THE NERD'S GUIDE TO PRE-ROUNDING: A MEDICAL STUDENT'S MANUAL FOR THE WARDS

This is a how-to guide for third-year medical students moving from the classroom to the clinical/hospital setting – a particularly stressful transition in a student-physician's career. This handbook is made up of short, easily digestible passages that advise students on everything from reading an ECG or chest x-ray to tips on dealing with ornery residents and what to wear on the wards. Passages are peppered with light-hearted anecdotes to bolster the spirits of students who may feel intimidated and overwhelmed by their responsibilities as fledgling doctors.

This handbook has been developed by Dr. Richard Loftus, who wrote the first version of this guide after his third year at UCSF School of Medicine. It began as a letter of advice to a junior student who was embarking on his own first year on the wards. As the author says of the first guide, "This covers everything I wish someone had warned me about before I stumbled onto the wards." This book contains appendixes of useful information, including links to full-size forms and data card templates that can be accessed at the Cambridge University Press website: www.cambridge.org/0521676754.

Richard A. Loftus, M.D., is an internist in private practice and a clinical instructor at the University of California, San Francisco (UCSF). A cum laude graduate of Yale College, he was editor-in-chief of the *Yale Herald*. After college, his work as an AIDS activist (noted in Jon Cohen's *Shot in the Dark*) and researcher led him to medical school. Upon graduation from UCSF School of Medicine in 2001, he was elected to Alpha Omega Alpha (medical honor society) and won the Gold-Headed Cane, the school's highest honor. That year he also won the UCSF Chancellor's Award for GLBT Leadership. He completed his residency in primary care medicine at UCSF, where he won both the Intern (2002) and Resident of the Year (2003) awards. In 2004 the students of UCSF School of Medicine recognized his devotion to medical education with a TEACH award, and UCSF Medical Center acknowledged his dedication to patient care with its Exceptional Physician award. He continues to teach students and residents at his private practice at Davies Medical Center, San Francisco, CA.

The Nerd's Guide to Pre-Rounding

A Medical Student's Manual for the Wards

RICHARD A. LOFTUS, M.D.

University of California, San Francisco

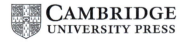

CAMBRIDGE
UNIVERSITY PRESS

CAMBRIDGE UNIVERSITY PRESS
Cambridge, New York, Melbourne, Madrid, Cape Town, Singapore, São Paulo

Cambridge University Press
40 West 20th Street, New York, NY 10011–4211, USA

www.cambridge.org
Information on this title: www.cambridge.org/9780521676755

First published 2006

Printed in the United States of America

A catalog record for this publication is available from the British Library.

Library of Congress Cataloging in Publication Data

The nerd's guide to pre-rounding : a medical student's manual for the wards /
Richard A. Loftus ... [et al.].
    p. ; cm.
Includes bibliographical references and index.
ISBN-13: 978-0-521-67675-5 (pbk.)
ISBN-10: 0-521-67675-4 (pbk.)
1. Clinical clerkship – Handbooks, manuals, etc.   2. Medical students – Handbooks,
manuals, etc.
[DNLM: 1. Students, Medical – Handbooks.   2. Clinical Competence – Handbooks.
3. Medical Staff, Hospital – organization & administration – Handbooks. W 49 N443
2006]   I. Loftus, Richard A.   II. Title.
R839.N47   2006
610'.71'1 – dc22   2005029452

ISBN-13   978-0-521-67675-5 paperback
ISBN-10   0-521-67675-4 paperback

Contents

Acknowledgments

These notes were generated based on my own experiences, as well as discussions and experiences shared with various peers. In particular, I'd like to thank Denise Albert-Grimaldo, Jim Ashe, Milana Boukhman, Fred Cirillo, Creighton Don, Leila Ettefagh, Kim Freeman, Marcel Gemperli, Stephanie Green, Eliza Humphreys, Ali Iranmanesh, Debbie Kahn, Tim Karaca, Ann Kim, Jae Kim, Naveen Kumar, Herprit Mahal, Matt Mazurek, Sharon Meieran, Steve Millar, Ginny Mommsen, Saam Morshed, Katie Murphy, Teri Onouye, Nora Osman, Alex Papanastassiou, Shanti Perkins, Karla Petersen, Nira Pollock, Debbie Rabitz, Ilya Reiter, Anne Rosenthal, Cynthia Salinas, David Schab, Michael Singer, Jody Stonehocker, Maya Strange, June Tester, Nhi-ha Trinh, Aslan Turer, Renee Ward, Elijah Wasson, Amy Whitaker, Lynne-Love Williams, Gillian Yeo, John Young, and Althaea Yronwode. I'd especially like to thank Jody Stonehocker and Denise Albert-Grimaldo, my role models on surgery and medicine, respectively. All of the above, directly or indirectly, gave suggestions or spurred ideas that have entered this document. I am grateful for their wisdom and for having shared various parts of my med school experiences with them. None of them, however, should be held responsible for any content in this text, and any mistakes, particularities, or editorial comments are solely my own.

I would also like to thank my many teachers over the past years, and especially Dan Lowenstein, whose knowledge, compassion, and sheer mensch-iness have been an enormous inspiration to me, and Meg Newman, for her endless support and kindness. I also want to thank my med school big sib, Britt Swor-Yim, and "adopted" sib, Gabriela Diaz-Sullivan, for always looking out for me, and my little sib, the most excellent Ted Scott, who is the reason I compiled these notes.

In Tibetan Buddhism, the practice of medicine and spiritual training are one and the same: All medical knowledge is ultimately attributed to the Buddha, in his form as Bhaisajyaguru, the Medicine Buddha. May every person pursuing the medical arts accumulate magnificent wisdom and endless compassion in the service of their patients.

OM BEKENZE BEKENZE MAHA BEKENZE BEKENZE RANDZA
SAMOUNGATE SOHA.

What Is *The Nerd's Guide?*

This book originally was written as an aid to medical students at the University of California, San Francisco (UCSF), during the start of their MS3 year, the first year of intensive clinical training. I wrote it at the end of my own MS3 year, based on notes I'd kept of all my "bonehead" moments. I made many errors that easily could have been avoided if I'd only known one or two simple facts. My feeling at the time was that despite excellent work by the UCSF School of Medicine in preparing us for the wards, there were still practical points that had not been covered ahead of time. I try to cover a few here.

The *Guide* is a starter kit to help MS3s "hit the ground running" during the first months of clerkships – especially for the inpatient months of medicine and surgery. There is nothing here that a thoughtful MS3 wouldn't eventually pick up on his or her own. The point of the *Guide* is to reduce the number of potholes in your road or at least make you aware of the common craters into which your predecessors have all too often strayed. Why repeat our mistakes, when you can make ones of your own? (That *is* a joke.)

Just as important as its practical tools for doing well on the wards, the *Guide* offers advice on how to maintain your well-being – physical, mental, and emotional – during the often-arduous trials of medical training. **The habits you develop during your student years will determine whether you thrive, or dive, during the rest of your career** – especially in the rigors of residency.

These habits include not only your approach to pre-rounding or reading a chest film, but also how you cope with stress, maintain morale, balance your checkbook, and exercise to keep fit. An alternate title for the *Guide* might have been *Advice From a Big Brother*.

The first version of the *Guide* was released in June 2000 as *The Nerd's Guide to Pre-Rounding: How to Look Smart While Feeling Stupid in the First Months of Third Year*. It was well received, so the following year I released an expanded Version 2.0, and the school asked for permission to post it on its website. I've since lost track of the number of students who have approached me on the wards, in the library, in elevators, all thanking me for the *Guide* (which was nice, but kinda weird). Older students give younger students their dog-eared copies. It appears to be useful.

I'm no expert on doing well on the wards and don't pretend to be. If anything, this book testifies to my proclivity for mistakes – after all, it grew out of my own errors. I have continued working on *The Nerd's Guide* based on feedback from UCSF MS3s that it has helped them. Errors in previous versions have been fixed as well, thanks to their remarks.

While this handbook evolved at UCSF, its advice about the approach to inpatient medicine would apply just as well at any academic medical center.

A final note: *The Nerd's Guide* is definitely **not** intended to be a comprehensive reference on surgical or medicine inpatient care. There are plenty of other books for that. The *Guide* instead serves as a "how-to" on the nuts and bolts of being a medical student, and how to do that job to the best of your ability – something other references don't usually cover. That said, you undoubtedly will use some of those other reference books in the months ahead – in fact, I recommend a few below.

Why is it called *The Nerd's Guide?* Because I'm a big nerd, that's why. (Well, technically, I'm a spazz, which is a subspecies of nerd, but now we're splitting hairs.) Seriously: I am a self-confessed medical "nerd" – I have the geek's love of details and the internist's delight in *obscurantia*. One of my first attendings told me she was worried my meticulousness would lead to early burnout. (Another ribbed me endlessly for a 4-page-long progress note I wrote on the differential diagnosis of a patient's fever.)

You don't have to be a Godzilla-nerd to benefit from the *Guide*. It will, however, give you some indication of what a thorough medical student's approach to inpatient medicine looks like. If some directives seem like overkill to you, well, at least you know where you stand. And if you feel totally clueless about starting on the wards – well, I'm with you. I *was* you. This *Guide* is designed to get you started, and not go too far wrong.

Tackling the wards. When you first start on the wards, your seniors will ask you repeatedly to do tasks you have never done before, and you may not know where to begin. If you're completely unclear of what you're supposed to do, a quick clarification ("So, you're asking me to do . . . ") is in order. If you understand the task, but don't know *how* to do it, find someone and ask them – ask your intern, ask a fellow student, ask a ward clerk or a nurse, hell, ask the janitor. Ask anyone. **Your attitude should be, "Well, no, I've never done this before. But I'll figure it out."**

When residents gripe about students, it's because students complain when they have to stay "late," or make remarks like, "I didn't think students had to do *that*." In my experience, no medical student has ever had to stay "late." "Late" is hour 37 of call, when you have not slept, and you've been in the ICU for the last 6 hours trying to keep a shock patient on *this* side of death's door. *That* is staying late, and it is not a condition students find themselves in until intern year. (Although, with the new work hour laws, hour 37 of call may also be a thing of the past . . .) Do NOT begrudge a resident who asks you to stay until 6 P.M. to finish an admission – or, I have to say, you'll deserve whatever he puts on your evaluation. **Ward work is teamwork. Pitch in.**

That said, **you should also expect to be treated with respect.** Everyone on the wards, from the attendings and patients, to the nurses and techs, to the medical and pharmacy students – all should be treated with humaneness and respect at all times. Moreover, while I feel students should be prepared to perform any service asked of them, you should **never do anything that violates your sense of safety or ethics.** (Such cases are fortunately rare; if you encounter one, bring it to your clerkship director immediately.)

There *is* a hierarchy on the wards, and it would be stupid not to acknowledge it. It exists because in life-and-death situations, experience counts. Period. While my anarchist political leanings make me suspicious of hierarchy in any flavor, I have developed a grudging respect for the pecking order on the wards. My advice: Don't tolerate abuse, toward anyone; but **students should submit humbly to the Chain of Being** (great or not so great, depending on your point of view). In the *Blue Beryl*, a fundamental text of Tibetan medicine, students are told to treat their teachers like gods, and to consider their wisdom like nectar. This may sound strange to the ears of autonomy-minded Americans, but I echo the sentiment. Even the scary hard-case attending may have something useful to teach you.

Finally, don't let what I've said increase your anxiety about your reception on the wards. The majority of residents and attendings welcome the addition of students to a team – for their assistance with the work, their enthusiasm, their curiosity, and, quite tellingly, their mostly intact empathy for patients, which can get ground out of people over the years. The students on my teams have demonstrated excellent knowledge bases, great clinical problem-solving skills, and (with few exceptions) great maturity and patient rapport. Expect to rock the house. Have confidence in yourself. (I do!)

And, in the tradition of *The Nerd's Guide*, I'd like to remind you, as you start on the wards, to consider your own ability to help your peers. Don't get distracted by the all-too-common delusions of ego and ambition that imbue our shared medical culture. They're bogus, and a trap.

Introduction to Version 1.0. *"I expected the third year of med school to be a tortuous test of will."*

And it has been, at times. Overall, though, I leave third year excited about my future medical career and amazed at the true privilege it is to take care of patients.

If you're like me, you will have many moments in third year when you will draw on knowledge earned with the sweat of the first two years. In terms of pathophysiology, biochemistry, pharmacology, clinical reasoning, etc., we are prepared. We have the knowledge.

However, we do not necessarily have the know-how. Knowing the branches of the internal carotid will not help you make an organized presentation in pre-rounds during the first week of clerkships. Knowing the up-regulators of glycolysis, or the sequence of drugs used to treat status epilepticus, will not help you get along with your team or get the evaluations you need to meet your career goals.

During the first day of each of my rotations, it was customary for the secretary of the clerkship program director to dispense a phonebook-thick stack of handouts intended to help "orient" us. I was often amazed at the gap between what they *thought* we needed to know and what we actually *needed* to know to function as medical students. **Our academic supervisors often tell us what they want us to learn, but not how we're supposed to do our jobs** – let alone how to do them well.

That is the reason for the following guidelines. These tips and suggestions are intended to help you "survive and thrive" during the intense early weeks of clerkship year. They are the kind of specific instructions I wished I'd had when I started third year. By halfway through the upcoming year, you will have learned on your own much of what's in this guide. But why stumble and learn things the hard way, when, with a little forewarning, you can look thoughtful and well-prepared?

A caveat: This is obviously a limited, and self-indulgent, first-person view of what will help you on the wards. **It's only my personal opinion**, but I offer it for what it's worth. – *RAL*

Dedication. The beginning of my internship in June 2001 was marked tragically by the loss of one of the most devoted clinical instructors UCSF School of Medicine has ever had: Dr. G. Thomas Evans, Jr. Tom's self-published *ECG Interpretation Cribsheets* was an indispensable aide for generations of UCSF students and residents. Just as important was his absolute commitment to the education of housestaff and his availability to us at all hours of the day and night. Tom's pure love of teaching, his cheeky irreverence, and his pursuit of excellence all were an inspiration to me. I miss him terribly. He exemplified qualities that I, too, esteem, and it is in this spirit that I dedicate this and all future versions of *The Nerd's Guide* to his memory.

* * *

Warning: Career Ahead

Before I even get into how to survive third year, a warning: It's over pretty fast. Before you know it, it's spring, third year's almost over, and you have to pick your sub-internships and get ready for applying to residencies. It sounds like it's far away, but it isn't.

There are three kinds of people going into clerkships:

- People who have a strong idea of what they want to do
- People who have a few options in mind, but no strong opinions
- People who have NO IDEA where they're going

Find an advisor. Or two. Regardless of which category you fall into, you will benefit from talking to someone who can advise you on reaching your career goal. Ideally, this would be someone working in your chosen (or prospective) field – a professor, a former preceptor, an attending you've worked with.

Notice I didn't say "mentor." The word "mentor" conjures the image of a god-like Mother-Father being, à la *Tuesdays with Morrie*: part Ward Cleaver, part Captain Kathryn Janeway, part Obi Wan Kenobi. Most students never find an advisor with this much benevolent parental mojo.[1] You can get great career advice

[1] Not that I have anything against mentorship. It's just that the term "mentor" gets thrown around a lot in situations where it doesn't really apply (sort of like "love" or "family values"). True mentoring is an organic relationship that grows out of circumstances – I don't think it can be planned or forced (as anyone whose college assigned them a canned, official "mentor" has probably learned). Since we're on the topic of mentors. . . there are usually two types of students: ones who have no

from normal mortals, and you don't have to meet with them every Tuesday of third year to get it. Even meeting twice might be enough.

Also, don't forget about your "big sibs" and senior students, who may be more helpful in sketching out your career terrain in the near-distance.

If you are a **"no idea" person**, it's harder to know where to start finding an advisor. I would say your **deans** are your best bet. Some schools, such as UCSF, have a formal system of "colleges" or "big sib networks" to help junior students meet senior students and faculty. For people without a strong direction, it's especially key to **start meeting with an advisor early** to get help on finding a career path. You might also consider reading a book such as Anita Taylor's *How to Choose a Medical Specialty*, or check **www.aamc.org/medcareers**. Make sure your third-year schedule gives you some broad exposure to various career options early on (i.e., before you have to pick your sub-internships).

People with a **strong idea** of what they're doing are released from the "Are you my mother?" agony that afflicts those looking for their niche. However, there are other issues. Again, your schedule should be arranged so you have a chance to try out your likeliest

---

mentors, and ones who have gobs of them. I am in the latter group, and if you're in the former group, I have some advice. Many of my mentor relationships evolved because I saw senior researchers or doctors at the medical center who seemed cool, and I would seek out ways to work with them (sometimes by arranging an elective; sometimes just by asking to meet with them). Big powerful folks don't always make the best mentors, since they have less time. Enthusiasm and energy are more important to me than a person's prestige, or even what they work on, although I tend to gravitate to people who share my interest in AIDS. Mentors should be thought of like nice outfits: You need different mentors for different occasions. I have "bench research" mentors, "clinical research" mentors, "academic career" mentors. . . . I have mentors totally outside my specialty. I even have "mentors in reserve" who I know I can seek out if I ever need advice on something I think they know well. Finally: The mentor relationship works both ways. It's like the old adage, "You have to be a friend to make a friend." People want to work with people with good energy and enthusiasm. Your success is *your* responsibility, not the mentor's. So, if you want mentoring: Go to the energy, collect mentors for different occasions, and remember that it's a two-way relationship.

choices earlier rather than later (again, before spring of third year).

If you're bound for a competitive specialty like radiology or dermatology, or a surgical subspecialty like ortho, urology, neurosurg, or the like, you may have to "shake the tree" a little to get exposure to the specialty early on. You should try to **find a mentor in the specialty early** to get help and advice. Your deans may be able to help you.

Finally, even if you know what you're going into, keep an open mind. You may find you love something you never would have considered. Think: "I'm going into Ob/Gyn – unless something else tempts me away."

Don't wait until the end of third year to think about career choices. You don't want to feel rushed when it's time to arrange a schedule. It's easy to be nearsighted during clerkships. Don't make that mistake.

* * *

The Job of the Medical Student

1. Get a thorough history.
2. Do a complete physical exam.
3. Make a concise presentation.
4. Write a timely progress note in the chart.
5. Do whatever is needed to learn about your patient and ensure her well-being.

If at any moment you get confused about your role on the wards or in the clinics: There it is. It's that simple. (Mind you, it may seem pretty intimidating at this point, but you **can** do it – even in the first week.)

In Appendix 3 I present "Patient Data Collection Cards," which include an initial history and physical examination record card. These should serve as informal "training wheels" you can keep handy while doing your H&P to ensure you don't miss any basic elements.

I also describe how to make a concise presentation – that is, how you'd summarize the daily update of your patient during routine bedside rounds (see Section V, "Pre-Rounding and Scut Basics").

The rest of your job. In addition, on inpatient services you will be expected to help your team with "**scut**," a term for "tasks related to patient care." Examples: calling a consultant, writing orders for labs or medications, doing procedures, getting the read on an x-ray. Interns do the bulk of the team scut but will often need your help to cover it all, especially on a busy service (again, see "Pre-Rounding and Scut Basics").

In surgery, you will also be expected to "assist" on operations. Mostly this means holding a retractor (referred to as "**water-skiing**" – if you don't get it, don't worry, you will) or suctioning blood or smoke produced by the "Bovey" (electric scalpel/cauterizer). If you're lucky, you will help suture.

You will also be asked to give "Presentations"[1] – either on your patient and her illness or on a special topic of interest to the team (see Section VIII, "Presentations: Here There Be Dragons").

What isn't your job. Your job is not necessarily to know up front the full differential for every presenting sign and symptom – but you *will* be expected to demonstrate your knowledge and, more specifically, that you have a systematic way of thinking about questions (see Section VII, "Pimping and the Art of Self-Defense"). This is not to say you shouldn't try to learn as many differential diagnoses as you can ahead of time, but to emphasize that you can still do a good job despite (temporarily) not having this knowledge.

Coping with "stage fright." If at any time you enter an exam room and think, "I don't know what the hell I'm doing in here," refer to the list at the beginning of this chapter. You don't have to think – just follow that list. If you feel **really** stumped, ask a fellow student, an intern, a resident, or an attending for help.

Once, when I went into an exam room, I found a patient who was there for follow-up of an elbow sprain. The first thing I thought was: "Hmm. I have no idea what's involved in evaluating this patient." If I'd only referred to the list above! Thanks to first and

[1] By the way, the word "presentation" is thrown around a lot, and deserves definition. There are several types of "presentation." On daily inpatient rounds, or in the clinic, you will be asked to "present" the patient – either a quick update on their daily progress or a quick summary of their history and physical. In addition to these "presentations," there are "Presentations," which last about 30 minutes (sometimes longer) and may involve looking up several articles on a topic or your patient's illness(es).

second year, I should have recalled that a patient with a limb injury should be checked for range of motion of the digits and for signs of nerve damage. A general physical would have also unveiled any additional injuries that needed attention, as well as other medical problems (that this patient had). All I had to do was 1) take the history, 2) do a full exam, and 3) present.

Bottom line: You have the knowledge to do at least the basic job. While it helps if you feel like you know the twelve different things that could cause your patient's symptoms, **you don't have to know all of what's going on to do your job**. Nor are you expected to know it all, at this point.

Your mission. Don't forget that, in addition to your "job," you have a mission: to learn as much as possible about the various areas of medicine to help you as you ascend in your level of responsibility for patient care. Even if you're not going to be a surgeon, you need to know how to recognize when your patient *needs* one.

No "boring" tasks or patients. I've noticed that most of our superiors, from attendings to interns, underestimate the role of "useless scut" as part of the educational experience. Presenting a patient to a consult service may be a "ten times a day" bore to an intern, but in your first months on the wards, it's a new activity. It probably *will* get boring to you after *you've* done it ten times. But initially, it's not a bore. So **be willing to help with scut**, and let your team know you're willing.

Likewise, you may notice that residents will characterize a case as "boring," as in: "Sorry you had to take the patient with the abscess – I wanted to give you something more interesting." Hmmm. How many abscess patients do they think you've cared for at this stage of the game? How many times have you done dressing changes, managed pain meds, or pulled housing out of thin air with the help of a savvy social worker? At this stage, it should all be fairly interesting.

* * *

Job Performance: The Big Ten

At most schools, clerkships use a basic set of criteria for evaluating student performance. Usually there are written remarks as well as specific grades for essential features of the student's role. At UCSF, grades are 1 (very poor), 2 (needs work), 3 (good but still can improve), and 4 (excellent). The ten features usually go something like:

1. Fund of knowledge/mechanisms of disease
2. History taking
3. Physical exam
4. Case presentations
5. Record keeping (progress notes)
6. Problem solving
7. Professionalism and responsibility
8. Self-improvement and adaptability
9. Relationships with patients
10. Relationships with teammates

Notice two through five? Those are your basic job description from Section II. One and six have to do with having medical knowledge and applying it. I can't help you there – but some advice may help you avoid coming off poorly when in fact you know your stuff. (See Sections VII through X.) Seven through ten mostly have to do with demonstrating that you care about doing a good job and using some emotional intelligence. Much of the advice herein applies to these evaluation criteria.

* * *

Gear Down: White Coats, Stethoscopes, and Other Fashion Accessories

So, what do you need to bring to the clinics and wards? I break gear down into three general categories:

1. Clothes
2. Tools
3. Books

Clothes: Whither the white coat? Rules vary by institution, but you can expect to wear the white coat on inpatient services, such as surgery, medicine, Ob/Gyn, peds, and surgical subspecialties. Often outpatient rotations – family, psych, and parts of peds and Ob/Gyn – will not require you to wear a white coat in the clinics, but you should have an ID badge or name tag displayed at all times. Even if clerkship directors don't require you to wear a white coat, it's prudent to wear one the first day rather than presume you don't need one. Make sure your coat is not too small – it should be loose, comfortable, and easy to get in and out of. (Note for when you purchase your coat: They often shrink in the wash, so buy in larger sizes.)

A practical advantage of the white coat is its pockets – perfect for carrying crucial books and other necessities.

Scrubs vs. regular clothes. On inpatient services, especially on-call, your superiors will usually be wearing scrubs. It's often convenient to change into scrubs early in the day – especially if later you'll be going to the OR. Thus, on such rotations you may not spend much time in "regular" clothes, and **while it's important to look nice, it's not necessary to invest in an extensive, pricey work wardrobe.** Still, if you're not in scrubs you should dress professionally.

A personal plug: I tend not to dress in scrubs unless I'm going into the OR or on-call and doing messy procedures. **While scrubs are practical, they can start looking sloppy** – especially after 24 hours. Patients deserve professional treatment, which means dressing nicely when it's not impractical. Dressing nicely shows a disciplined exterior, which hopefully reflects/encourages a disciplined interior. Part of looking smart is looking smart.

This also goes for outpatient services. Dress as you would for a formal occasion – meaning, something you'd wear to a friend's wedding (except for the shoes, ladies). As I say to my medical students: "The hospital is the Temple of Healing, so dress in your Sunday best." (Or Saturday best, depending...)

Shoes. There are two schools of thought. Some invest $100 in a good pair of shoes; others go cheap, or don't bother with special shoes at all.

I'm normally a cheapskate, but I belong to the first group. I think it's wise to **invest in a comfortable pair of shoes** – you'll be wearing them constantly. In my class, many went with clogs for inpatient services. One student said she found it painful to spend that much money on shoes, but she has never regretted her decision. In fact, she now finds it painful to wear any shoes besides her clogs! (We will not digress into a discussion of "clog addiction" at this time.) For men, I recommend Ecco brand. They're expensive as hell, but they look great, and they're like walking on air. Despite long hours on my feet, I've never once been distracted by foot pain.

Other students bought inexpensive loafer-type shoes. One student bought no new shoes and wore her tennis shoes on surgery and dress shoes for other rotations. To my knowledge, shoe purchases have had *no* bearing on evaluations.[1]

Tools: The black bag. You'll need something in which to carry your tools and books. Some people put everything in their white coat pockets. Others use a small bag, mini-duffel, or similar item. At UCSF, many people use a small hiking fanny pack. Now, what to put in it?

You may be surprised to learn that medical students often act as the "caddy" of the team – which means **your residents and attending often will not have their tools and expect to borrow yours.**

Every medical student should always carry:
- Stethoscope.[2]
- Pen light.
- Reflex hammer – although in a pinch the edge of your scope's diaphragm will work.
- 2–3 spare black ink pens – your superiors will often steal yours!
- Alcohol wipes – for wiping your scope's bell between patients. Bugs are transmitted by dirty tools. If you're going to wash your hands, wash your scope.

On inpatient rotations, it's also convenient to have:
- Surgical shears.
- Tape – "Micropore" paper tape is the most versatile; other types may be too strong/sticky for human skin. You can "borrow" from the supply room.

---

[1] I have heard from admission committee members, however, that shoe selection *has* been raised in discussing prospective applicants to UCSF medical school. Don't you find that flabbergasting? (Makes you wonder if the right clothing purchase will make you a "shoe-in" for admission. Sorry, couldn't help the pun.)

[2] You may consider attaching a stopwatch to the end of your scope, or at least keeping one handy. I don't know about you, but I have a hard time estimating a minute, or even ten seconds, when counting a heart rate. If an attending asks you to check the pulse, having a watch handy makes estimating the heart rate during auscultation much easier.

For the slightly nerdy:
- Small tape measure – giving exact measurements of lesions/ locations looks smart.
- Hemocult guaiac[3] cards and developer – because you can never find it when you need it.
- Snellen test vision card – if you want to test CN2, especially on inpatient services.
- (Small) travel alarm clock – more reliable for waking up on call nights than the wimpy "alarm" function on most pagers; recommended.

Usually not needed:
- Tuning fork – might be good to have in locker for new admits if neuro issues are at play.
- Other neuro exam tools – as above.
- Oto-opthalmoscope – store in your (locked!) locker during inpatient rotations, since most rooms don't have them; out- patient clinics usually have one.
- Spare bandages ("Four by Fours," "Two by Fours" – no, they're not lumber) – you can get these from a supply room before rounds, if needed.

Needed only for international rotations to the Antarctic:
- Blood pressure cuff/sphygmomanometer.

By the way: **Label your tools.** There's not that much variety, and people's gear can get mixed up. Also, attendings will borrow your stuff, walk off with it, and then not remember which med student they took it from.

Books. We'll cover other texts below, but there are a few little reference books you will want to keep on your person.

---

[3] Pronounced "GWEYE-ack."

Every medical student should always carry:

1. *Tarascon Pocket Pharmacopoeia* – I used it 20 times a day.
2. A basic handbook. I recommend the *Hospitalist Handbook*, Sanjiv J. Shah, editor, UCSF Department of Medicine. This little gem can be purchased from the UCSF bookstore (phone 1-800-846-2144). Even then, it may be tough to get a copy. Fortunately, it is on-line at http://medicine.ucsf.edu/housestaff/ handbook/index.html. A PDA version can be downloaded, and there is an outpatient guide as well. Another popular hard-copy choice is *Pocket Medicine: The Massachusetts General Hospital Handbook of Internal Medicine* by Marc S. Sabatine. These are compact, all-purpose references, highly practical, and helpful even on non–internal medicine rotations.
3. A peripheral brain – see Section VI.

For the slightly nerdy:

4. *The Sanford Guide to Antimicrobial Therapy* – I used this maybe once a week.

Other useful references (not necessarily needed on your person all the time):

5. An ECG interpretation book. There are literally dozens. *Rapid Interpretation of EKG's*, by Dale Dubin, is a great basic reference. It is produced by Cover Publishing Company (Tampa, FL). More information is available at Dr. Dubin's website, www.themdsite.com/permissions.cfm. Another easy-to-carry basic ECG guide is the *Pocket Guide to 12-Lead ECG Interpretation*, by Gerry C. Mulholland (Baltimore: Lippincott Williams Wilkins). Once you've mastered the basics, I'd like to give a plug for the tiny but highly practical *ECG Interpretation Cribsheets*, by G. Thomas Evans Jr., M.D. Tom was the Jedi Master of ECG reading at UCSF. His reference is excellent but has a convoluted organization not appropriate for the complete novice. Appendix 1 contains a basic approach to the ECG. Once

you understand the basics, the Evans book can take you further. You can order it via the UCSF bookstore: www.bookstore.ucsf.edu/pg_evanscribsheets.html.

Usually not needed on your person:
6. Fred Ferri's *Practical Guide for the Care of Medical Patient* (St. Louis: Mosby)
7. *Washington Manual* (Boston: Little, Brown and Company)
8. "Baby" *Harrison's*, etc.

They're just too darn big, and you don't usually need them at a moment's notice. They are helpful to keep in a locker for study and reference. If you find something in them you'd like to have on your person, xerox it and slap it in your peripheral brain – or, these days, get the PDA version and load into your handheld.

* * *

SECTION V

Pre-Rounding and Scut Basics

What's "pre-rounding"? What's "rounds"? For inpatient services, most of the planning and work on patients gets done before 10 A.M. "Rounds" refers to visiting, literally or figuratively, each patient on your team's service. There are several flavors of rounds. After **pre-rounding** to collect information on your patient, you and your team meet up for "**work rounds,**" which is where the resident is informed by students and interns about the state of the patients. This can last a couple of hours, if it's a large service and you're going room to room. Following work rounds often is "**attending rounds,**" a similar affair in which the patients are presented to the attending. (Sometimes there are no attending rounds, and the resident meets privately with the attending to "**card flip**" on the patients, which allows the team to do their work.)[1]

A presentation at rounds involves summarizing the patient's findings, analyzing problems, and describing an action plan for the rest of the day. The format for a work rounds presentation is described in the next pages. For attending rounds, you usually skip the "S" and "O" and just give a brief version of "E" and the "A/P," but otherwise it's similar.

---

[1] Another type of rounds is "**grand rounds**" – educational lectures given by a professor or attending. In the old days these, too, were given at the bedsides of patients, and were extemporaneous. Modern-day grand rounds share little in common with the old-style rounds, other than the name.

To be ready for rounds, there must be a "pre-rounds." This is when you, the medical student, gather your data, plan your presentation, and begin to write your note (a more detailed text version of what you present). By the way: Your note should be done as soon as possible, ideally by noon.

The time to begin pre-rounding depends on the service and when rounds will start. For a medical student, I advise giving yourself at least 30 minutes for each patient you're covering (usually one or two at the beginning of the year.)

Now, what to do? Pre-rounding tasks are listed below. They are in rough chronological order. They are also, arguably, in order of priority:

1. Get the vitals.

2. Examine the patient.

3. Get the labs.

4. Check the medications record.

5. Talk to the nurse.

I recommend using cards to record the data from these steps. On the following page is an example Patient Data Card. Appendix 3 contains an actual template.

Example Pre-Rounding Patient Data Card

MS3 Progress Note							
Date:	HD/POD:			Abx:			Diet:
							IVF:
Events overnight:							
Subjective:							
Objective:							
Vitals:	Tm	Tc	BP	P	RR	SaO2	
I/O's:	po + ng/gt + IV / uop + stool + emesis/NGT + CT						
24-hr fluid balance:							
Medications:							
PE: Chest:							
Heart:							
Abd:							
Wound:							
IV lines, tubes, drains:							
Labs:							
Studies:							
A/P:							

It's easiest for me to review the methods of pre-rounding by explaining the progress note. Next to the note, you can see what a student would actually say on rounds, versus what's written on their note.

Data	How you'd present it on rounds
HD/POD: Hospital day/Post-op day. Example: "3/2"	"Mr. Jones is our abscess patient.[2] He's hospital day 3, post-op day 2."
Abx: Antibiotics. Keep track of total days patient has received antibiotic treatment, as well as the number of days of each of the specific drugs they're on. (Patients sometimes start one drug, then switch.) Example: "cefazolin #2, 1 g IV q8hrs"	"cefazolin day 2."
Diet: Patients waiting for a procedure or with certain disorders like pancreatitis will be "NPO" – nothing by mouth. Other possibilities would be: "regular," "ADA" (American Diabetes Association), "clears,""soft," etc.	"He's on clears but still feeling nauseated post-surgery, so he's on D5-1/2 normal saline plus 20 milliequivalents KCl, 100 cc's per hour."
IVF: See Appendix 1, Fluid basics	
Events: Basically, anything significant that's happened to the patient since the last report – usually, "no events." Other events could be "Patient spiked a temp overnight," "had fits of vomiting," "complained of dizziness," etc. Depends on the case.	"No events overnight."

---

[2] If this were a patient the team had not heard about before, or it was the student's first time presenting him, they might want a "bullet," or summary on who he is. For example: "Mr. Jones is a 54-year-old postal worker with suppurative hidradenitis. He presented with an abscess of the right axilla that required incision and drainage." Medicine teams might want more PMH in the bullet, but in general, short is good.

Data	How you'd present it on rounds
Subjective: What the patient has to say about his or her condition. I usually record exactly what they say, in quotes. Usually things like, "I feel okay," or "My pain is worse and 8/10," or "Couldn't sleep last night." If you want a specific question for this, ask about pain.	"Says he slept okay but is still nauseated."
Objective: Vitals: It's best to record the last set of vitals, usually found on a clipboard on the bed or outside the room. You should also record the range of values over the past 24 hrs. T_m = max temp in 24 hrs; T_c = current temp; BP = blood pressure; P = pulse; RR = respiratory rate; Sao_2 = oxygen saturation, which should be expressed as percent and under what conditions, e.g., "99% RA" or "99% on room air," "94%-2L NC" or "94% on oxygen by nasal canula, rate 2 liters/min."	"He's afebrile, vital signs stable[3]."
I/Os = Ins and Outs. A record of fluids and substances in and out over 24 hours. P. O. = by mouth; ng/gt = nasogastric/gastric tube; UOP = urinary output; CT = chest tube. You should note the fluid balance per day and since admission.	"He's had 2.6 liters in, 2.4 IV and 0.2 by mouth. He's had 2.4 liters urinary output, and had 2 bowel movements. He's down 0.2 L for yesterday but up 0.3 since admission."

---

[3] You can also report "T_m 37.5" vs. "afebrile," since a T_m below 38.5 indicates patient has no fever. Teams will usually appreciate the brevity of "vital signs stable," but, early on, your resident may want you to report the vitals. If so, it's best to give a range over the past 24 hours, rather than just the most recent set. Example: "Blood pressure was 115–135 over 70–85, pulse was 60–82, respiratory rate was 22, sat was 99% on room air."

Data	How you'd present it on rounds

Meds: I think it's a good habit to check that patients received their meds. Some wards have a "med book" that you can check to see what your patient got, and when. I would put this in the note, but *only rarely* present – if so, as at the right→

"He got his Kefzol as ordered. He's had 2 mgs of morphine at 15 and 23:00 hours, and he just got 2 more 20 minutes ago in preparation for wound packing, which we'll do shortly.[4]"

PE: Physical exam. The basic pre-round exam should be very quick and has five parts. Traditionally, most people check the chest, heart, and abdomen. If the patient has a dressed wound, check to see if it's "C/D/I" – "clean, dry, intact." I suggest also inspecting the IV – make sure it's not inflitrated or shows signs of infection.[5] Also check other tubes or drains to make sure they're open and don't show signs of infection. The normal chest exam is recorded as "CTAB" – "Clear to auscultation bilaterally." The heart is "RRR-no MRG" – "regular rate and rhythm, no murmurs, rubs, or gallops." Abd: "BS +, S, ND/NT" – "bowel sounds were present, abdomen was soft, non-distended,[6] non-tender." I would then report on the wound condition, if appropriate. You can record the IVs or tubes in the note, but don't present them unless there's a problem.

"On exam, the chest was clear to auscultation bilaterally, the heart had regular rate and rhythm, no murmurs noted, and on the abdominal exam, bowel sounds were present, abdomen was soft, non-distended, and non-tender. Wound dressing on right axilla was clean, dry, and intact, with packing wick evident under the bandage."

---

[4] Pearl: Changing wound packing in I&D (incision and drainage) surgical wounds *hurts*. Call the nurse when you start rounds and have her give a morphine dose about 15 minutes before you change the packing.

[5] By the way, peripheral IVs should be changed after 4 days, 3 if placed in the ER; usually the nurses take care of this. See Appendix 1, "Admitting a Patient/Meg's List," for more info.

[6] Bowel sounds "present," never "positive."

Data	How you'd present it on rounds
Labs: Recording these is pretty straightforward. Traditionally, they're recorded in the following order: CBC (WBC, Hgb, HCT, platelets); "lytes" (Na, K, Cl, HCO3, BUN, Cr, gluc); note the anion gap, if any; "LFTs" or liver panel (AST, ALT, T bili, alk phos); "Coags" (PT, INR, PTT); Ca/Mg/ Phos; other labs (amylase, lipase, albumin, etc.). You don't have to announce the test and then its value for CBC or lytes, just announce the panel – they know what numbers are what if you go in correct order. Also, you don't have to indicate if values are high or low – teams usually know what's normal or not. Record whether numbers are trending up or down on the progress note. You may indicate in rounds, depending on the case.	"CBC was 9.8, H&H[7] 14, 42, platelets 220. That white count's down from 11 yesterday. Lytes were 140, 4, 100, 25, 15, and 1, with a glucose of 72. In short, Mr. Jones is a 54-year-old man with suppurative hidradenitis, 2 days status-post incision, and drainage of a right axillary abscess. Overall, doing very well. His issues include:
	1. Wound. So far, healing well, no pus. We'll continue daily packing changes.
	2. Infection. He's afebrile 24 hours, with white count down. We'll check the CBC today, but it looks like the Kefzol's working, so we'll continue it.
Studies: Tip: For urinalysis, give pH, spec grav, then the pertinent + and −'s.	3. Pain. Adequately controlled with morphine. We'll need to wean him to TyCo3s for discharge and will start today.
A/P: Assessment and plan. This is the most important section of the presentation, and the point at which most students choke. Suggestions on how to go about constructing this section are outlined next.	4. Nausea. Could be post-general anaesthesia, or due to the morphine. We'll try starting him on Compazine today and see if it helps.
	5. FEN. As I said, I'd like to get his nausea under control so he can increase his po's. Then we can d/c the IV, maybe this evening if he's better.
	6. Prophylaxis. He has Ted hose; on docusate.
	7. Dispo. To home when clear. Probably tomorrow, if he remains afebrile another 24 hours.[8]
	8. Code status: Full code."

[7] "H&H" = hemoglobin and hematocrit.

[8] Traditionally, patients must be afebrile (T <38.5°C) for 48 hours before discharge.

Tips on rounds presenting. *"Think like Dickens, speak like Hemingway."* In other words, know all the details, but don't say them all. Knowing how to edit yourself is an acquired skill you will pick up over time, so don't worry if you're a tad confused about what to include/exclude in your rounds presentation. The rule of thumb is that **short is better.** In fact, the longer the list of patients on your service, the less commentary and analysis you should give – in the above, for example, we might not break down the ins and outs into the various types of fluid, just "2.6 in, 2.4 out, up 0.3 since admission." And in our A&P, we might eschew the assessment of the problems and simply give the plan: "Nausea. Will start prochlorperazine." If the attending or resident wants more from you, they will ask for it. (Which means you should have it ready.)

To create an assessment and plan. First, you should give a global assessment. The example repeated Mr. Jones's name, age, diagnosis, and hospital course. It also gave a global assessment: "Doing very well." Other descriptors could have been "stable," "recovering slowly," or "seems worse," etc.

Then give the problem list, with an assessment and a plan for each item. To create a problem list, it's helpful to think in terms of all the issues that have arisen on the patient. Some services, especially intensive care units, like to organize problem items by organ system, e.g., "1. Neurologic function, blah blah. 2. Respiratory, blah blah." On most services, however, problem items should be specific problems, not organ systems. Notice in the Jones example, some items were diseases (wound or infection) and others were symptoms (pain and nausea). What constitutes a unique problem item is a subjective call. In a patient with ESRD (end-stage renal disease) and hyperkalemia (K), docs who are "splitters" might number each of those as separate issues (one chronic, the other acute), whereas "lumpers" would put them as one problem, since the K problem is due to the ESRD. Splitting tends to be more thorough and is a better approach for students at the beginning.

Almost always, the first problem is the one that brought the patient into the hospital. The remainder should be presented in order of urgency – what poses the greatest danger to the patient's health, will keep her in the hospital, or is her greatest concern. Rounding out the list will be some other routine items described below. *Most of the following items should be considered once – upon admission to the hospital – but some should be thought about every day (although not actually mentioned in rounds).* The mnemonic is **"FEN, 8P's, and D/C"**:

- **FEN** = "fluids, electrolytes, nutrition." You should review what's going on in this category daily, because problems that arise in this category can be catastrophic and usually occur because no one was paying attention to them. Mr. Jones is not really getting much nutrition by mouth, due to his nausea (problem 4). Fortunately, he hasn't developed any electrolyte problems. If he had, we might comment on them here or make them a separate problem item – e.g., "problem two, hyponatremia."[9]

- **Pain.** Any day your patient reports pain should be a day you place "pain" on your problem list. You may have already addressed pain as part of the treatment plan for the patient's main problem(s) on admission, but if you haven't, thinking of it as a separate item will ensure you don't forget to treat ALL of their sources of pain. For example, a diabetic presenting with chest pain may have long-standing neuropathy pain as well, and may already be on a routine outpatient medicine for this. Often you just have to ensure they continue to get their regular medications – especially if those include opioids.

Besides "treat *all* their pain," a second basic principle is to switch patients to oral pain medicines as soon as circumstances allow – patients cannot go home with an IV.

---

[9] The causes and management of common electrolyte disturbances are covered in the *Hospitalist Handbook* of the UCSF Department of Medicine (available at http://medicine.ucsf.edu/housestaff/handbook/index.html).

PRN pain meds. Most patients will have a **routine** PRN order for "acetaminophen, 650 mg po q4hrs PRN fever/pain." If other acetaminophen-containing medicines are written for the patient, you should specify that "acetaminophen dose not to exceed 4 g/day." Patients with liver disease should have an order to limit acetaminophen to 2 g/day. (Note that acetaminophen in low doses is often safer than NSAIDs, even for liver patients.[10])

It's often good policy to have a PRN order for **breakthrough** pain as well. For most patients, a typical order might be "morphine sulfate, 2–4 mg IV q2–4hrs PRN breakthrough pain, hold for sedation or RR <10." All patients written for opioids should have PRN orders for docusate and senna (see Appendix 1).

Ongoing pain. Patients with continuous pain should be ordered for a long-acting pain medicine and something for breakthrough pain. Determining the correct dose of a long-acting pain medicine usually is done by writing the patient for breakthrough IV pain meds, then totaling the dose they required for a 24-hour period and converting it to a more convenient oral medicine (see Appendix 1). **Patients with pain should always have a breakthrough pain medication order,** in addition to their basic or long-acting pain medication coverage.

PCAs. Patients with significant pain syndromes – e.g., sickle cell patients with a pain crisis – may be more appropriate for "patient-controlled analgesia," which is an IV pump that supplies medication at a slow basal rate. The pump has a button the patient can push to deliver a breakthrough dose when needed. Pumps are programmed to limit the total number of breakthrough doses, so as to avoid an overdose and suppression of respiration. A PCA can reduce pressure on the nurses to respond to repeated requests for breakthrough pain doses and can improve total pain control.

---

[10] Riley, TR 3rd, Bhatti, AM. Preventive strategies in chronic liver disease: Part I. Alcohol, vaccines, toxic medications and supplements, diet and exercise. *Am Fam Physician.* 2001;64:1555–1560. Erratum in: *Am Fam Physician.* 2002;65:2438.

Special note on chronic pain and methadone patients. Keep in mind that patients on methadone or long-acting high-dose opioids (e.g., sustained-release morphine or oxycodone) will go into withdrawal if you neglect to write for these meds. This category includes injection drug users (IDUs) who shoot heroin – they have a high tolerance for opioids and need higher doses of pain medicines than patients not regularly exposed to opioids. (IDUs may need to be placed on methadone maintenance while in the hospital.) Ask your residents for guidance.

- **Prophylaxis.** There are many forms of "prophylaxis" on inpatient care. Four big ones:
  1. **Stress ulcers prevention.** A common issue, especially in surgery patients, many of whom receive cimetidine or other H_2 blockers for this purpose. Conventionally, indications for anti-stress ulcer prophylaxis include having a coagulopathy, being on a vent for >48 hrs, having a previous history of a GI bleed, or having certain special problems (burns, liver failure) while in the ICU.[11] **Most ICU patients should have ulcer prevention.**

     Supposedly, sucralfate is a better choice for gastritis prevention than is cimetidine for patients on ventilators, because the former is less associated with pneumonia. This is controversial, however.[12] The controversy is likely beside the point, since these days we usually use proton pump inhibitors. We don't know if PPIs pose the same risk for patients who aspirate as do the H_2 blockers. We do know that for most uses, except for patients who have

[11] Lam NP, Le PD, Crawford SY, Patel S. National survey of stress ulcer prophylaxis. *Crit Care Med.* 1999;27:98–103.

[12] Kappstein I, Schulgen G, Friedrich T, et al. Incidence of pneumonia in mechanically ventilated patients treated with sucralfate or cimetidine as prophylaxis for stress bleeding: bacterial colonization of the stomach. 1991;91:125S–131S. See also Driks MR, Craven DE, Celli BR, et al. Nosocomial pneumonia in intubated patients given sucralfate as compared with antacids or histamine type 2 blockers. The role of gastric colonization. *N Engl J Med.* 1987;317:1376–1382.

an acute upper GI bleed (in whom PPIs have proven better in multiple studies), **H₂ blockers and PPIs are equivalent.**[13]

That said, **if your patient doesn't have an indication for stress ulcer prevention, don't give it.** It won't help and it may harm.

2. **DVT prevention.** Risk factors for deep venous thrombosis in hospitalized patients include obesity, immobility caused by travel or orthopedic surgery, malignancy, previous DVT, age >40, recent MI, having lupus anticoagulant, having varicose veins, pregnancy, oral contraceptives or hormone replacement, and having inheritable pro-coaguable conditions such as Factor V Leiden, a common mutant clotting factor.[14] There are several preventive measures. One is getting up and **walking.** There are also **"Teds and SCDs"** (Ted hoses are anti-embolic stockings that fit snugly around the legs; SCDs, pronounced "scuds," are "sequential compression devices" – balloon-like trousers that squeeze alternate locations around the leg[15]). Finally, there are anti-coagulant drugs, like **heparin or enoxaparin.** A common order would be "heparin, 5000 units SQ q12hrs."

   Unlike with ulcer prevention, I tend to err on the side of giving DVT prophylaxis. If you can think of a good reason why you're not giving heparin or at least compression stockings (e.g., the patient is active and walking the halls every day), you can hold off.

3. **Constipation prevention.** During my first week as an intern at Moffitt Hospital, I had a patient who didn't have a bowel movement for a week. She became obstipated, perforated

---

[13] Cash, BD. Evidence-based medicine as it applies to acid suppression in the hospitalized patient. *Crit Care Med.* 2002;(6 Suppl):S373–S378. Review.

[14] Kimmerly WS, Sellers KD, Deitcher SR. Graduate surgical trainee attitudes toward postoperative thromboprophylaxis. *South Med J.* 1999;92:790–794.

[15] The anti-embolic effect of SCDs is not dependent on their location – in fact, a SCD attached to an arm has just as much benefit. The squeezing of the veins appears to release some sort of humoral anti-clotting factor.

her colon, and was rushed to the ICU in shock. You should know the date of your patient's last BM; **no one should go more than 3 days without a BM.** Most patients warrant automatic bowel regimens, since they're often bedbound and thus stool less often. I usually write: "Docusate, 250 mg po BID, hold for loose stools," and "Senna, 2 tabs po q12hrs PRN constipation, hold for loose stools." You may also use bisacodyl, 10 mg po q12hrs, or other cathartics, in place of senna. If the patient doesn't respond to routine cathartics, convince yourself they're not obstructed (i.e., benign abdominal exam, looks well, passing gas) and then try a Fleet© or tap water enema. The "secret weapon" that almost always works is "Lactulose, 30 cc po q2hrs until BM." It's unpleasant, but will work. If you induce diarrhea this way, make sure to check electrolytes afterward.

4. **Medicolegal events prevention.** Poor communication is a major factor in most medicolegal events. Establishing a plan for communicating with patients and their families will go a long way toward reducing the chances that a medical problem will turn into a legal problem for your team and the hospital. Phrased more positively, good communication greatly enhances patient satisfaction. This can be as simple as **taking down the family's phone number at admission** and asking them to leave messages for you at the nurses' station, which you can return at your leisure. Bedside rounds should usually end by asking the patient, **"Can we answer any other questions or concerns?"**

   Personally, I err on the side of copious availability, especially in the case of patients who are critically ill or have a terminal illness. I often give families my pager and ask for their indulgence of my sometimes-delayed replies. (Note: Some programs may ask you NOT to give out your pager number; if so, you may prefer to direct calls to a voicemail or e-mail account, as an alternate way for families to reach you.) I may have to explain that I prefer channeling communication through one family member, since my schedule makes multiple phone calls impossible. Most families have an obvious point person or can designate one. I usually ask for a cell phone (best choice), or dual home and work numbers.

Having contact info will help you in many ways, not the least of which is the last-minute disposition of a patient thanks to having the business number of the family member who can come to pick them up.

- **Precautions.** I would not review this as a daily category, but consider it the first time you compose a problem list for a patient on admission, or if their status changes. Common categories include:

1. **Aspiration precautions** (for patients with altered mental status, new stroke, severe dementia, etc.). This involves, for example, nurses keeping the head of the bed elevated >30 degrees. Such patients may need supervised feeding of a special diet (e.g., thick liquids).

2. **Falls precautions** (again, frail elderly and the like). For nurses, this means keeping bedside rails up, assisting patient in getting out of bed, perhaps only allowing urination into a container, etc. While nurses may be inclined to ask you to write for physical restraints for such patients (e.g., to keep confused patients in bed so they don't get up and inadvertently hurt themselves), there is no evidence that such restraints prevent injury – indeed, restraints have been known to result in injury and death. Alternatives to restraints may include moving the patient close to the nurses' station, ordering a "low bed" flush with the floor (so they don't have far to fall), and even music therapy.

3. **Seizure precautions** (if seizure history, or alcohol withdrawal with a seizure history). Again, this is mainly giving nurses a heads up. If the patient has seized recently, you may also want to request "Yanker suction device at

bedside," so you can quickly suction their airway if they seize again.

4. **Sensory deficits** (e.g., blind on one side or deaf). The need to flag this for nurses should be self-evident.
5. **Neutropenic precautions** involve limiting access to the patient's room, no fresh flowers or produce, etc. You may need to specify "neutropenic diet." For patients with <500 absolute neutrophil count.

Precautions should be mentioned once on the first A&P list and should be entered into the nursing instructions on the admit orders.

- **"PRNs."** This is covered only on admission. These are medications written to be given as needed. Examples:

1. "Acetaminophen, 650 mg po q4–6hrs PRN pain or fever."
2. A "sleeper" med. For people under 60 years, "diphenhydramine, 25–50 mg po q bedtime PRN insomnia." (Note: You can also write this as "PRN insomnia or itching," and make it a two-for-one.) For very sick or older patients, avoid anticholinergics, since they can cause altered mental status. Thus, for them: "trazodone, 25–50 mg po q bedtime PRN insomnia." Do not write sleepers for patients who are confused. Otherwise, virtually all patients deserve a sleeper med – sleeping in the hospital is close to impossible. Indeed, my mentor Dr. Michelle Roland writes them as an automatic medication; e.g.: "trazodone, 25 mg po q bedtime, patient may refuse."

Those are the most important PRNs. Other common ones include "diphenhydramine, 25 mg po q6hrs PRN itching" (caution with elderly or very ill); "magnesium/aluminum hydroxide, 20 ml po q4hrs PRN heartburn" (caution in renal failure – magnesium may accumulate, watch lytes if they're using it); and "simethicone, 40–125 mg po q6hrs PRN gas/bloating."

- **Prerequisite tests.** This is an item to review at admission only. It mostly applies to patients accepted direct to the floor, who may not have had common baseline tests often done in the ED. Of course, some patients may not get all needed baseline tests even when they *do* come through the ED. Specifically, consider whether your patient needs a baseline ECG CXR (chest x-ray), and/or UA (urinalysis).

You don't always have to order such tests, but having baseline studies can be helpful. One example: I had a patient with leukemia who developed hypoxia and tachycardia. Worried about a pulmonary embolus (PE), I checked an ECG and found he had incomplete right bundle branch block (RBBB) – which can be a sign of PE. Unfortunately, he'd been accepted as a transfer on a busy call day, and we never got a baseline ECG; it was unclear if this RBBB pattern was new or old. A baseline ECG for comparison would have helped a lot in his assessment.

- **"PT/OT."** Like prophylaxis, this may not be something you mention each day, but it should be on your mental list of A&P items to think about. PT/OT stands for "physical therapy/ occupational therapy," which is appropriate for many patients who have lost function or stand to lose function while convalescing in the hospital – e.g., post-surgery, post-stroke, frail elderly. (There is more on rehabilitation services, and do's and don't's of working with them; see Section X.) On daily rounds, this problem item could be presented as simply as, "Number 8, PT and OT are seeing the patient." I usually mention it right before prophylaxis, dispo, and code.
- **"Psychosocial."** This could be higher on the list in a patient who is, for example, expressing extreme anxiety or depression, or has been disruptive with staff. I think you should always have an idea of what the patient's psychosocial condition is, but as with precautions, you should not mention it unless you feel the team needs to intervene.

- **"Primary."** As in, someone should be designated to call the patient's primary care provider sometime in the first 24–48 hrs to let them know of the admission. Usually the resident does it, but it should be discussed (*briefly*) as a problem item on admission, to clarify who's going to take care of it.
- **"Dispo."** Meaning, disposition. In other words, the plan for discharge. Typically, "To home when clear." If the patient doesn't have a home, or may not be safe at home (frail elderly), then a social worker needs to be consulted to sort out a plan with you, the patient, and/or his family. See Appendix 2, "Dispo Dancing."
- **"CODE."** Meaning, the patient's code status. **Code status should _always_ be your last problem item and _should be present at the end of every note._** If your patient has an event overnight, the team on call will check your note to confirm the current code status. Code options include "full code," "DNR" ("Do not resuscitate"), and statuses in between. See Appendix 6, "Eliciting the Code Status."

Now what? Once you have a list of problems, break each item out according to (1) diagnostic issues and (2) treatment issues. (On outpatient services you add a third: patient education.) For each issue, think in terms of "assessment – how this has evolved since admission," and "plan – where we're going."

For example, in the case of Mr. Jones's infection (problem item #2), it was noted that he'd been afebrile for 24 hours and WBC was down (diagnosis – assessment), and that the team was getting another CBC today, presumably to follow his white count (diagnosis – plan). It was noted that the cefazolin antibiotic seemed to be working (treatment – assessment) and would be continued (treatment – plan).

For new problems or symptoms, it's appropriate for the "diagnosis – assessment" to briefly describe the possible causes of the problem, that is to say, a differential diagnosis. See problem #4, nausea, as a short example. Your assessment should ideally indicate what is the likely cause, since it might affect the choice of proper treatment. In the Jones example, while morphine was mentioned as a cause of nausea, there was no plan made to stop or switch the drug – which implies that the presenter didn't think this a likely explanation.

In truth, there are almost as many ways to create an assessment and plan as there are doctors. Hopefully, my approach gives you a framework for making a problem list and presentation. Your residents can give you more instruction when you hit the wards.

Just a final note on pre-rounding: The last of the five tasks I mentioned at the start of the chapter was "talk to the nurse." If the patient is groggy, the nurse will be able to discuss any overnight events of which you should be aware. Also, if any questions have come up while reviewing the other documents – e.g., apparently missing doses of pain meds or antibiotics, vitals not recorded, IV removed and no note in the chart about it – she or he can probably answer them.

Always reserve 10 minutes of pre-round time at the end to figure out your assessment and plan for each problem. It's also a good idea to practice your presentation, at least mentally.

Once you present, listen carefully to the team discussion about each problem and note down any "to-do" items you hear. After rounds, talk to your intern about the "scut list" for your patient, and ask her which ones she wants you to do. I find it helpful to create a to-do checklist next to each problem item on my card, on my scut sheet, or in my progress note.

Scut – how to prioritize it. After all the patients on the service have been presented, there will be time to attack the scut or to-do items for your patient. **Taking care of scut is the responsibility of the interns, but they often rely on medical students to help out** and will delegate some scut to you. As an MS3, you'll rarely have more than two or three patients to cover, at least at first (although this is institution-dependent). As an MS4, you may have as many as six or seven, sometimes more on a heavy service, and you're on your own (although your R2 will help you).

At the end of the section, I've attached a sample "scut sheet" as a tool to prioritize your scut. I use actual copies of this sheet each day on the wards to help me stay organized. This is crucial, because time is limited, the work can seem endless, and some scut items are more important than others.

The scut sheet[16] is designed for a clipboard. Each row indicates a patient, and patients are listed from the bottom of the page upward, **starting with the sickest patients** (usually in the ICU), followed by less sick (transitional care – not in the unit, but high-level nursing care), followed by regular floor patients, usually clumped together by location, i.e., patients all on the same floor listed together.

Each column is a type of scut item. Items to the left have higher priority and should be done first, followed by items in the next column, etc.

Calling a consult. You'll notice **calling consults** is done first. Examples include calling infectious disease service to get advice on the choice of antibiotics or calling renal to help assess a patient in acute renal failure. **As a general rule, you should contact the consult team before noon,** unless the patient happens to get sick and needs urgent attention late in the day. Fellows expect to hear about new cases as early as possible.

Some fellows and consult attendings refuse to take calls from medical students. This is not rudeness – just an impatience with student ignorance. If your resident asks you to call a consult service, you must ensure you can **state precisely what question you are asking.** If it's not self-evident to you, it will not be self-evident to the consultant. Also, ask your resident if she wants to

---

[16] For a downloadable version, go to: www.cambridge.org/0521676754.

hear back from the consultant with a phone call or if she just wants to check the note in the chart later.

Be prepared to give the consultant a mini-presentation about the patient. This includes basic information such as patient name, medical record number, and location; your team's attending and resident and their pager numbers; most recent vitals and lab values; and background information, such as an abbreviated version of the initial history and physical and the main events of the hospital course to date. **Have all of this information at your fingertips *before* you call.**

Once you've explained the nature of the consult and given the basic information, and the consultant confirms that he will see the patient, **find out when the team can expect to hear back** regarding impressions. I often finished the conversation with, "Thanks. And in case my resident asks me, can you tell me when you think you might have recommendations for us?"

Other scut. After consults, the next item is **ordering[17] studies,** e.g., x-rays or CT scans. The sooner these are ordered, the more likely the patient will actually get them that day.

The next item is **"D/C."** If the patient is being discharged today, filling out discharge forms and discharge prescriptions takes priority – and may, in fact, trump ordering studies on other patients. Patients who are within a day or two of discharge should also be flagged – **as a medical student, you will help your intern**

---

[17] On writing orders: Usually, medical students can write orders, but they must be co-signed by a resident or attending. Order writing is learned from your seniors as you do it. It's helpful to keep patients' charts handy during bedside rounds so that someone (who is not presenting) can write down orders as the team decides on them. Prepared students keep blank copies of order sheets for their patient so that if they think of orders they can write them out and have their seniors co-sign them immediately, rather than having to go fetch the chart. (For hospitals with computerized orders, this is obviously unnecessary.) For the first year of writing medication orders, check them against your pharmacopeia for proper dose and frequency, every time. This section of *The Nerd's Guide* includes many examples of common orders, which you can use as guides when writing orders on your own.

a lot by filling out discharge paperwork a day or two early. Some patients will have special social work needs prior to discharge, and those should be undertaken at least a couple of days prior to discharge.

Note that routine orders are given lower priority than items already described, but you can often get them out of the way during rounds if you keep the patient chart nearby when you present. As soon as a plan is agreed on, write the orders. This takes care of scut before it even *becomes* scut.

After orders, the next item is "**Check . . . ,**" as in "Check to make sure PT has started seeing patient," or "Check on why patient didn't get chest x-ray last night" – i.e., troubleshooting. This is followed by **calls** to services other than consult services – e.g., social work – and then **miscellaneous scut.** This latter category often includes non-urgent procedures, which are usually done after lunch and after most other scut is completed.

Also, each row has a little checkbox next to the patient's name to mark off when the daily note has been finished. Notes should, in an ideal world, be done by noon.

The final column is "**Sign Out.**" This may not be pertinent for MS3s, but MS4s leaving the hospital will be responsible for "signing out" their patients to the cross-covering intern who is on call that night (see Appendix 5, "The Don't-Panic Pages: For the Sub-I"). During the day, key items that need to be brought to the attention of the cross-cover during sign out can be jotted down in the last column.

Warning: The main point with organizing scut is to be as fast and efficient and possible – **don't be so rigid in prioritizing that it slows you down. Be flexible.** Scut should be prioritized based on the needs of the patients, and in some cases a patient may be sick enough that you spend all morning on his needs and defer the rest of the patients' scut (except maybe consults) to the afternoon.

Name, ward	Consults	Studies	D/C?	Orders	Check...	Calls	Misc	Sign Out
□ note								
□ note								
□ note								
□ note								
□ note								

Date:

* * *

Knowledge Management: If I Only Had a Brain . . .

THE CLERKSHIP BINDER

I recommend bringing an empty binder to the first day of each clerkship for storing the various documents you will be handed by your clerkship director's administrative assistant. Mine has sections for "Schedules" (for daily rounds, conferences, call assignments, etc.), "Presentations and Write-Ups," "Computer Info," "Academic Objectives" (such as crib sheets for the exam or the list of what's on the exam), "Key References," and "Misc." Keep it in your locker or backpack.

There are at least two reasons to do this: (1) The mass of paper can bury you; sorting it in a binder helps you get on top of it, which makes it helpful rather than a hindrance. That way you can find what you need when you need it. (2) You never know when a random question about "Which student is on call tonight?" or "Is breast surgery going to be on the exam?" will come up. If you keep the stuff piled under your desk at home, it's not going to help you when you need it.

THE PERIPHERAL BRAIN

Every student should start one of these on the first day of clerkships, in my humble opinion. Most residents and even attendings have their own peripheral brains; if you get started building one now, it'll be that much more complete when you get to that level.

At this point, I use my PB nearly every day. Also: I noticed that **my medicine residents were very impressed that I already had a PB** (despite its relatively scant content). They decided I was smart and meticulous – an impression that may not have been true, but which certainly helped me. So, start building a brain, if for no other reason than that **it makes you look conscientious,** which will help you on evaluations.

What it is: In the pre-PDA days, my PB was a small (6″) soft-bound binder with loose-leaf paper. (Now I keep it as a set of memos in my PDA; you can use standard memo format, or a note-taking program such as ThoughtManager™ by HandsHigh Software.) The PB is a customized set of organized notes and "cheat sheets" of information you can't quite commit to memory and that you use all the time. For example, the inside front cover of mine has a list of commonly used emergency resources for patients (emergency shelters, etc.), and the inside back cover has a table of routine weights and measures as well as metric/English conversion formulae.

My first page (after a cover page with my name and phone numbers) is a list of **normal lab test values,** such as you get at the front of a typical exam. I've written them using **those funky shorthand diagrams,** such as "the fish" diagram, which is used for electrolytes.

```
 Na  | Cl   | BUN    /
-----+------+-----< Glu
 K   | HCO3 | Cr     \
```

This helped me to remember which values were for which test when I encountered a note like this:

```
 140 | 100  | 15     /
-----+------+-----< 85
 4.0 | 25   | 1.0    \
```

I recommend asking about these "shorthand" diagrams during your orientation "information management" session. The special shorthand diagrams for other tests include:

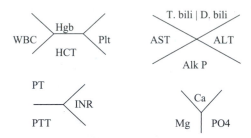

How to organize it. The rest of my PB is organized alphabetically by medical and surgical specialties – a section for cardiology (diagnosis and treatment of acute MI, how to read an ECG, etc.), endocrine (diabetes, hyperparathyroidism, etc.), infectious disease (HIV, endocarditis, etc.), neuro (stroke, seizure management, etc.), ortho, etc. I also have a section on "Procedures" and on "Pharmacology." The latter contains little pearls related to specific drugs or groups of drugs.

Especially important (for me) is another section on "Problem-based diagnosis." In this section, I have notes on how to work up a presenting complaint, e.g., Chest Pain, Leg Pain, Shoulder Pain, Fever, Shortness of Breath. **Developing differential diagnoses of symptoms or signs is a major task of third year,** and having notes on presenting problems will help you to do this.

Thanks to endless numbers of grand rounds, formal clerkship seminars, and informal teaching on the clinics and wards, you will easily be able to fill your brain by year's end. **Make sure you jot down the article reference or name of the person from whom you got the information, so you can look it up again if the information is ever questioned.**

By the way, the PB also lets you record administrative information, such as **your login and password codes** for various hospital computer systems. You may obtain such codes at one hospital, then forget about them, only to need them again when you return to that hospital months (or even years) later. Put them in your "brain." *Then* forget them. Until you need them again.

How your PB can make you look like a mega-genius. Personal testimony: After finishing surgery, and following a pancreatitis patient, I had a nifty little section on the diagnosis and management of pancreatitis. Later, on my medicine clerkship, we admitted a lady with pancreatitis. Now, in the U.S., most cases of pancreatitis are due to alcohol or gallstones. This lady had neither in her history. While my residents were scratching their heads, trying to figure out why she had pancreatitis, I looked at the other causes of pancreatitis in my PB notes. Under one of the other causes, "medications," I had written "thiazides, steroids, tetracycline." And I realized that this lady had been on tetracycline for a sinus infection. So, there was our likely suspect. And I piped up: "Hey, she was on tetracycline, that can cause pancreatitis!" And I looked way smart. You, too, can pull off stunts like these, and ace your clerkships, simply by building a brain.

CARDS: KNOW WHEN TO HOLD 'EM

Patient data cards are a common method for keeping track of important information on patients you're following in the hospital. Many students at UCSF use a version of the **Patient Data Collection Cards** (see Appendix 3). Students usually copy the forms onto colored card stock. The first card is an initial history and physical card, which by tradition is tan. Lab values are recorded over time on a yellow card. Daily exam, vitals, and problem listing is included on blue cards – enough of these to cover the hospital course. Residents, whose information templates are already in their heads, usually use blank index cards. I recommend using pre-formatted cards of some kind as **training wheels** until you get comfortable with the sorts of data you need to follow on your patients.

There are various philosophies about using patient data cards. **Some residents don't like students using cards, because they think it's inefficient for students to write down information twice:** once on their cards and then again on their progress notes. They advocate writing pre-rounding data on a blank progress note, once. (If you do that, make a copy of the note to keep on your person for reference before entering the note in the chart.) I support using the cards, at least at first, since that was how I learned what to put on a progress note in the first place. Cards may be helpful at hospitals with computerized charts, where there are no blank paper progress notes to keep on you during pre-rounding. If you use cards, you can **also carry blank progress notes during pre-rounding,** and try to record pre-round data on the progress note during rounds. This will make it easier to get notes finished by noon.

Be forewarned that **some attendings hate students reading off their cards** during rounds. I actually had an attending and resident grab my card set out of my hands and command me to present without my notes. (Was this incredibly patronizing? Yes, it was. Did it piss me off? Yes, it did. However, I was able to present perfectly well without the cards. For more commentary on such incidents, and how to handle them, see "The Horrible Truth About the Wards" in Section IX.) To the best of your ability, you should try to present without looking at your progress note or "daily note" card, but I think it's okay to refer to your card when reporting exact vitals or exact lab values.

By the way: **label your card set**. Use a key chain with a tag on it, don't just put your name on one of the cards – no one who finds a lost card set is going to tab through the cards looking for the one with your name on it. Until you get used to carrying a card set, you may occasionally misplace it. If you put a name tag on it with your pager number, a kindhearted nurse or tech who finds them can call you and get it back to you. Otherwise, you may take a long time to find it, or never find it and have to rebuild from scratch. Quite a pain. I misplaced my cards three times during third year, and the second two times I was called within the hour by someone who happened to find them.

USEFUL REFERENCES

I'm not going to go into an exhaustive account of all the books I used on the wards. Just a few tips:

1. ***Sapira's Art and Science of Bedside Diagnosis***. By Jane M. Orient (Philadelphia: Lippincott Williams & Wilkins, 2000). If you desire to improve your physical exam skills, **get this book**. *Bates* is to *Sapira's* as *See Spot Run* is to *The Brothers Karamazov*. An endless trove of clinical exam tips and pearls. Go from physical exam "dud" to "stud" in 600 pages.

2. **A problem-based diagnosis book.** Patients do not usually enter your care with the chief complaint, "Doctor, please help me, I have new-onset congestive heart failure." They say, "I feel short of breath lately, especially at night." Rather than resorting to *Current Medical Diagnosis and Treatment* – which would require that I *knew* what my patient had – I often referred to *Problem-Oriented Medical Diagnosis* by H. Harold Friedman (Baltimore: Lippincott Williams & Wilkins). The *Ferri's Clinical Advisor* (St. Louis: C. V. Mosby) apparently has a problem-oriented section, which some students have recommended. It's worth finding and keeping a problem-based text around, especially in third year, when the diagnosis for a patient's sign or symptom is not obvious.

3. **The Yale Wards Handbook**. Yale School of Medicine has an on-line, student-written handbook for the wards. It has a separate section of tips for each rotation, from surgery to medicine to Ob/Gyn. I used some of these and they were very helpful. Find them at: http://info.med.yale.edu/osa/wardshandbook/index.html.

4. **An on-line reference.** The on-line reference UptoDate (www.uptodate.com) is an invaluable resource for the areas of medicine, family practice, Ob/Gyn, and peds. Many medical centers have institutional accounts that students can use. If you are not fortunate enough to be in such a place, I would strongly consider the substantial investment in a personal account (currently $195 for medical trainees with proof of trainee status; group rates may be negotiated for several purchasers). The

advantage to having an account is that you will have thousands of pages of organized, easy-to-understand references on medical subjects available via any web-worthy computer. In late 2004, a similar product called www.CMDTonline.com was launched, with lower prices and a free 30-day trial. Another excellent resource, whose registration is often free to students, is **emedicine.com**. And, for high-quality teaching materials on rapidly evolving topics, such as HIV/AIDS, **medscape.com** is another free and excellent on-line resource.

5. *Surgery Recall*. (Blackbourne L, et al. Baltimore: Lippincott Williams & Wilkins.) Awesome. Saved my butt multiple times. Also written by students, for students. I don't know about the other books in the "Recall" series, but this one is worth its weight in gold. By the way: Surgery attendings have caught on to students using this book, and they badmouth it. (I think they're mad that it's taken away their pimping advantage.) DON'T get caught reading this book – you risk a tirade from an ornery surgeon. But use it.

6. *Harrison's* vs. *Current Medical Diagnosis and Treatment*. Now, I have to confess, I have a sentimental soft spot for *Harrison's Principles of Internal Medicine* (Kasper DL, et al. New York: McGraw-Hill), and keep the 14th edition by my bedside. *However*, real-world experience has shown that *Current Medical Diagnosis and Treatment* (Tierney LM, et al. New York: McGraw-Hill/Lange Medical Books) is much easier to use. I recommend it. And in the interest of full disclosure: Many of the authors of *CMDT* are faculty and mentors of mine – but I recommended this book well before I met or worked with any of them.

BEING PREPARED FOR SPECIFIC MEDICAL CASES

The review file. I recommend, as much as possible, collecting a handful of review articles on common problems likely to be seen during your particular rotation ahead of time and keeping them in a binder in your locker for quick reference. The on-line Yale Ward Handbook can give you a list of "hot topics" for particular rotations, as can any specialty-specific textbook, e.g., *OB/GYN Secrets*, *Handbook of Pediatrics*, etc.

Why do this? It may help you a lot. Personal testimony: I kept a set of such articles, including one on the management of acute stroke, for medicine. One call day, my intern flagged me and said, "Meet me in the ER in 15 minutes. We're admitting a patient. I think it's stroke." Aha! So, I went to my locker, pulled out an excellent review from *American Family Physician* on stroke management, and read up. When I went down to the ER, I was able to make a couple of solid suggestions for managing the patient – including points that my intern wasn't even aware of! Which made me look way smart.

Obviously, you can't do this for every problem. But if you pick, say, five things that are likely to come up, you may have a chance to "sneak a peek" at a crucial moment – before heading down to the ER for the admit, before the impromptu teaching session at attending rounds, etc. – and wind up coming off very well. Even if at breakfast that very morning you wouldn't have been able to spell the diagnosis, much less explain it.

If you have an on-line reference account such as UpToDate, you may be able to run a quick search on the pertinent topic ahead of time, making a hardcopy review file unnecessary.

Creating a review file requires comfortable use of Medline, often accessed through PubMed (www.pubmed.com). If you're not comfortable with it, find a friend who is and get tutored. The more you practice using PubMed, the better you get. Meanwhile, I have some tips about using PubMed in Appendix 8.

PAGER ETIQUETTE

Many medical centers have specific protocols, or "pager etiquette," for sending pages. At UCSF, when we page someone we punch in the call-back number, star, and then our personal pager number. The latter allows the recipient to know who's paging him, and, if he's delayed in calling you back, he can page you later. When I was paged the first time on the wards, I was baffled by receiving two numbers: I didn't know which to call. Text pagers will eventually circumvent such problems.

Also, some centers may develop pager codes for other purposes. For example, at UCSF, "2222" first meant "come to the second floor," the location of the cafeteria – i.e., "time for dinner." These days "2222" simply means "food's here," even if the team ordered out.

Some services will have free pagers for medical students to use during the rotation, but frankly, I'd say it's more convenient to get your own personal pager and use that – that way you don't have to learn a new piece of hardware every time you change services.

Finally, it may go without saying, but if you place a call to a pager, know whom you're paging (or whom you're *trying* to page), and have your question or information ready (see Section V, "Calling a Consult").

PERSONAL DIGITAL ASSISTANTS (PDAs)

By 2001, more than 20% of all M.D.s used handheld computers,[1] and at this time probably the majority of students use PalmPilots™, Visors™, or the like on the wards. The use of a PDA is now assumed for most health professionals; residents transfer notes on them, references come in digital formats, etc. I would advise buying one as soon as possible if you don't already have one.

I'm afraid of my toaster, do I need a PDA? Yes. But don't be afraid. The American Medical Student Association has a nifty overview article about PDA basics on its site (www.amsa.org/resource/pda.cfm). The EctopicBrain website (http://pbrain.hypermart.net/basics.html) also has a collection of articles on getting started and frequently asked questions.

---

[1] Chasin MS. How a palm-top computer can help you at the point of care. *Family Practice Management.* 2001; 8:50. See also: Lewis M. Evidence-based-medicine tools for your palm-top computer. *Family Practice Management.* 2003; 10:73. These articles are available online.

What programs do I need? I think most people find benefit from having a medical calculator, for sure, such as SkyScape's Archimedes™; a general medical reference, such as *Harrison's*™ or *The Washington Manual*®; a drug interactions program; a document-reading program; and some sort of personalized note-taking program, such as HandsHigh's ThoughtManager™. Depending on circumstances, programs such as a medical Spanish dictionary may also come in handy. The take-away point is that **you can get many of the tools you need for free** and don't have to spend a ton on software.

Your peers are often your best source of information about useful software, but several websites can give you some tips. Matthew Delaney's article (www.palmsource.com/interests/education_medical) lists useful free software programs for medical students, including Epocrates® and McGraw-Hill's Diagnosaurus™, and includes a link to his website for downloading freeware (www.geocities.com/docpanama). Dr. Kent Willyard also gives a nice overview of various programs for distinct purposes (medical reference, medical calculator), with his remarks (www.palmsource.com/interests/medicine).

WHAT ABOUT HIPAA?

The Health Insurance Portability and Accountability Act of 1996 governs, among other issues, the disclosure of so-called protected health information (PHI), which is essentially any medical information attached to any identifiers such as name, medical record number, and Social Security number. Every institution is responsible for dictating how it complies with HIPAA, and each institution that you rotate through will likely have some sort of "How We Handle HIPAA" training for you. Like most health providers, students use PDAs and often record what would be considered PHI onto them. Individual worksites have different rules about such activity, but as a general rule, **if you keep any patient-related data on a PDA, you are obligated by law to protect your PDA with a pass code,** so that if it is stolen no one would easily have

access to the data. Likewise, remember that whenever you syn-
chronize your PDA with a computer, the PHI is transferred, and
the same security concerns apply – i.e., your computer should
have a pass code so that passersby or thieves cannot easily access
any PHI that happens to be on your machine. Again, different institutions have different guidelines on this. The American
Association of Medical Colleges has posted an article address-
ing other aspects of HIPAA as it pertains to medical students
(www.aamc.org/members/gir/hipaa/aamchipaafaqs.pdf).

The hazards of PDAs: They can go on the blink and throw
your day into chaos. They can also be misplaced. Or simply stolen.
While I know applications like PatientKeeper™ were in vogue for
a few "rapid adapters," at least at one point in time, here's my two
cents: Replacing a set of lost paper cards is much cheaper – and,
given that cards are often less laborious to use, may be faster for
many purposes. You can drop card sets on the dirty hospital floor
a hundred times, and while they may look crummy, they are still
as useful as before. PDAs are not quite so resilient.

* * *

Pimping and the Art of Self-Defense

"Pimping" refers to superiors asking a med student "on-the-spot" questions to see if they paid attention in the first two years of school. Many students hate to be pimped, since it makes them feel, well, on the spot. If you don't know something off the top of your head, you feel (even if you don't look) stupid.

1. **Have a method.** The key to pimping is this: While it's good to be able to give the particular answers your pimper is looking for, often what they want to see is that you **have a systematic approach to thinking about a problem**. Sometimes, even if you don't know a patient's particular diagnosis, showing you have an approach to the problem will earn you credit. I've often proceeded to give a particular diagnosis as an answer, only to have the resident stop me and ask for a broader differential.

Let's take the following example:

ATTENDING: What do you think of your patient's shortness of breath?
STUDENT: (Ulp!).... Well, uh... It's due to her congestive heart failure... (I guess...)
ATTENDING: Is that all?
STUDENT: Um... Well, that's what she has! I mean, I guess she could have pneumonia...

Better approach:

ATTENDING: What do you think of your patient's shortness of breath?

STUDENT: Well, I know our patient has CHF, which can cause this. But in general, when I think of shortness of breath, first I think of *lung-related* problems. Problems in the lung that could cause dyspnea could be *infectious*, such as pneumonia or empyema … Or could be *vascular*, such as an embolism … Or could be due to a *cancer*, or other space-occupying lesion … Or *surgical trauma*, causing a pneumothorax. There's also *cardiac-related* problems that could cause shortness of breath, such as congestive heart failure leading to pulmonary edema. … There could be a *hematological* cause, like anemia …

This latter example combines two approaches to creating a differential: the organ- or system-based approach and the etiological approach. The latter style can be summarized with the mnemonic "CHOPPED MINTS," which stands for Congenital, Heme, Organ failure, Pregnant, Psych, Environmental, Drugs, Metabolic-endocrine, Infection, Neoplasm, Trauma, Surgery-iatrogenic.

This advice may not apply to every situation, but keep it in mind. Attendings have a stereotyped idea of what med students should know, and **they often expect you to give answers in terms of mechanisms of disease, NOT specific diagnoses.**

2. **Be ready.** Read up on as many of your patient's problems as possible before you encounter a resident or attending. Use the Ferri manual or a similar quick reference. If you're going into the OR, review the basic anatomy and nature of the procedure beforehand (*Surgery Recall* is an excellent resource for such ad hoc reviewing).

   During my surgery rotation, an unfortunate student (*not* from UCSF) went into the OR without even knowing what surgery was being performed. BAD IDEA! When he caught a glimpse of a vessel, he blurted out, "Is that the aorta?" WORSE IDEA! This was a popliteal bypass – he was looking at the patient's knee! Ouch! The attending screamed, "Get him out of here!" (Not a very civilized reaction to a hapless student's faux pas, but not surprising.) I suppose that's one way to avoid getting pimped in the surgery suite . . .

Many schools emphasize giving students protected time, so they can read and study. USE THE TIME. Be ready.

By the way: *JAMA* ran an essay about pimping many years ago.[1] The piece is a satire advising young attendings on the best way to intimidate students and house officers with inane questions. It offers some funny, if not practical, examples of how students avoid answering tough questions – and how attendings can counteract these countermeasures. Weirdly, most of the letters written in response to the essay apparently took it seriously and critiqued its historical inaccuracies; questioned the legitimacy of the word "pimping," which doesn't appear in any English dictionary; and castigated the author for promoting a practice that has a negative effect on morale. (!) Guys, lighten up!

[1] Brancati FL. The art of pimping. *JAMA*. 1989;262(1):89–90. Replies in *JAMA*. 1989;262(18):2541–2542.

* * *

SECTION VIII

Presentations: "Here There Be Dragons"

As mentioned, there are "presentations," day-to-day brief summaries of patients you're following in the hospital or have just seen in clinic, and then there are "Presentations," which are usually the student's "spotlight moment" to show their stuff and garner a good evaluation. A Presentation is usually a grandiose version of the first time you present the patient, summarizing their entire H&P, the differential of their presenting problem, and the workup yielding the final diagnosis. (For the ultimate examples of a case presentation, see the *New England Journal of Medicine*'s "Case Records of the Massachusetts General Hospital" series – there's a case in almost every issue.) The Presentation may include a mini-lecture on a topic related to the patient's case. Sometimes the Presentation will not cover the H&P at all and will simply be the mini-lecture on a chosen topic.

When you give a specially prepared Presentation on a patient, here's a warning: **The Presentation may not be on the subject you think it is.** Both I and a classmate had experiences of preparing talks on special subjects related to our patients – in my case, various methods for imaging metastases in colon cancer patients, and in his case, drugs for treating PCP.

Both of us were horrified to find ourselves shanghaied by attendings who pimped us on aspects of the case we weren't prepared to talk about. In my own case, the attending stopped me in the middle of my talk and started pimping me about atrial fibrillation – a cardiac problem that had emerged as a postsurgical complication but had nothing to do with his reason for surgery. I confess, at that moment I recalled almost zero about a-fib, other than that it was an arrhythmia often seen in old folks that was often tolerated just fine with treatment. That's it. That's all I knew. I didn't even know the ECG pattern associated with it.

Well, needless to say, I started feeling like *I* was getting a-fib by the time my attending had asked her fifth or sixth cardiac-related question. Finally she stopped, looked at me, and said, "Didn't you learn ANYTHING in medical school?" (Sigh.... Again, unnecessarily deflating treatment from a superior officer: uncivilized, but unsurprising. See "The Horrible Truth About the Wards," in Section IX.)

How to deal with this? **Know the basics on every item in your patient's problem list, not just their main diagnosis. Also know the basics on all of their drugs – including the rationale for using them for your patient.** This way, if your attending turns your Presentation into a "hostile interview," you won't look *completely* lost.

Oh, another warning about Presentations: You may slave away on an assigned talk only to find the attending has totally forgotten about it, or there isn't time to present it at the scheduled time. This happens very often, more than the above scenario. If this happens, **resist the temptation to burst into tears** or tell off your resident. It's not personal; it's the way of the wards. You will likely have a chance, eventually, to give it, so keep the materials handy. Often, just as soon as you've totally forgotten about it, your senior will say, "Hey, weren't you going to give us a talk on __? Why don't you give it to us now?"

It's okay to assertively remind your team or attending if you have a Presentation that's overdue. If the time passes and you've shown due diligence, but there simply wasn't time for you to present, well...chalk it up as a learning experience. Save the handouts – you may get a chance to give the talk to a different group at a later date.

* * *

Making the Grade: Emotional Intelligence Trumps All

At UCSF, clerkships begin the onset of formal grading. Many of us, reverting to lifelong habit, focused our anxieties in terms of getting good evaluations, which are seen as the key to reaching career goals. While a solid fund of knowledge is usually the first item on the evaluation scorecard, I maintain that **emotional intelligence may ultimately play an equal or greater part in your evaluations as your strict competence or knowledge.** Some students may be completely oblivious to this reality, to their peril.

By "emotional intelligence," I mean things like your adaptability, maturity, sense of humor, professionalism, and ability to get along with others. Such factors are also part of your "scorecard" – however, they have a stronger global influence on your evaluators than other single characteristics.

Take, for example, my comments about carrying a peripheral brain. Although I'm not a slouch in the fund of knowledge department, I am usually pretty spazzy when pimped and often come off a little clueless. However, the fact that I carried a peripheral brain showed a professionalism that prejudiced my superiors in my favor. As a result, I think they often "upgraded" my "fund-of-knowledge" score, despite the fact that my knowledge base may have been pretty average. This is an example of **how professionalism can positively impact other characteristics of your performance.**

The following comments are intended to help you be ready for the environment of the wards and clinics so that you can demonstrate professionalism, even under duress. They are also intended to give you a gut sense of what sorts of demeanors, attitudes, or behaviors come off well on the wards.

THE HORRIBLE TRUTH ABOUT THE WARDS

They are very different from the "kinder, gentler" environment of the medical school. Many students are mildly traumatized when they witness, or receive, grossly rude or disrespectful behavior on the part of their superior officers. The humane and respectful treatment students receive in preclinical years may contrast sharply with the too-often toxic and disrespectful treatment on the wards.

How to deal with this? I recommend, first of all, that you prepare ahead of time for such conditions, so that you are not surprised when you see/experience beastly behavior. A little ego trouncing is de rigeur for students on the wards. In fact, **your ego on the wards is like carry-on luggage on a plane trip: If it's too big, it's going to get smooshed.** You're better off not carrying it with you.

I think it would also be a good idea to remember how it feels to be treated that way, so that you will not perpetuate such toxicity when you (in short order) ascend the ranks of power. Personally, I'm baffled as to why behavior that would never be tolerated in any other work environment is simply ignored in our own profession. Only our collective resolve to eliminate such behavior, or at least not perpetuate it, will improve conditions for those coming in our wake.

A sense of humor is crucial. It's also important not to take rude treatment personally – usually it has nothing to do with you and virtually any medical student in your shoes would be receiving the same treatment. Talking over experiences with your classmates, and venting, are also great releases. **And if you wind up in a bathroom stall crying, that does not make you a loser.** You are in very good company – you'd be surprised at how many of us have literally been in that place. It is a healthy sign that you are a human being, with feelings. Allow yourself the right to feel hurt. And remember the problem is with a medical culture that tolerates such unprofessional behavior, not with you.[1]

Meanwhile, here's a weird idea: It's called "**empathizing up.**" As students, we're often encouraged to put ourselves in the place of our patients and empathize with their needs. Since Western medicine is traditionally hierarchical,[2] with patients on the "bottom rung," I call this "empathizing down." However, we're rarely instructed to put ourselves in the role of our superiors. Yet our residents and attendings may be suffering almost as much, emotionally, as our patients. They are overworked, underpaid, exhausted, and often don't see their loved ones for days at a time. They may have lost marriages, relationships, and other cherished parts of their lives to their careers. None of this is an excuse for bad behavior, but **when someone behaves toxically on the wards or clinics, keep in mind that they probably are not malicious – they're just thoughtless.** They may just be having a bad day (or a bad life!). Their bad behavior is an outgrowth of their suffering. If you keep that in mind, you may forget about how bad you felt being on the receiving end of their cattle prod, and instead develop compassion for someone in a bad place – or at least a resolution not to repeat their example.

When working with "toxic" personalities, I try to focus on some good characteristic of the person. I assume everyone I work with on the wards has something to teach me. This helps me find ways of working with them. That grouchy resident may be an excellent team leader. Or, as one of my peers commented, "Dr. Jones *did* make me cry when I presented to him – but he also coached me and taught me how to make a good presentation."

---

[1] Why do students elicit such treatment? A quick analysis: Most doctors tend to be perfectionist control freaks, and many of them are secretly insecure. Seeing students stumble reminds them of their own personal development as doctors and of their own shortfalls. The way they treat their juniors, especially students, is a projection of their own neurotic insecurity and self-denigration.

[2] Not that I endorse this.

Also, don't be too quick to label someone as a "bad guy." If your intern is post-call the first time you meet her, she may not be the person she usually is with the team. So don't rush to judge. I found it usually took a week for me to a get a measure of a person.

Being able to bounce back from bad treatment with humor and maturity will always help you. In fact, at times it may make a crucial difference in your evaluations. So, aim for it.

Also: While you may need to tolerate some "rough treatment," you should never put up with treatment you consider abusive – especially if you feel sexually harassed, or if you feel personally attacked. In such cases, it is professional, and responsible, to report it to your program director.

VITAMIN C; OR, "YOU SHALL FEAR NEITHER RHINO NOR TIGER"

If I could give one piece of advice on how to do well on the wards, this is it: "*Conduct yourself at all times with cheerful confidence.*" That's it. People who always seem confident always do well on the wards, even if they have only so-so funds of knowledge and patient skills. Ask any fourth year, and they'll confirm this. It's startling.

By the way, some people confuse "projecting confidence" with "having a big ego." This is incorrect. It is possible to outwardly *seem* confident while inwardly feeling unsure. It is your demeanor that is important. Think about the old campaign for Arid antiperspirant: "**Never let 'em see you sweat.**"

Now I, unfortunately, was not someone who could pretend to feel confident, or cheerful, when I had utterly no idea what was going on and was worried sick about looking stupid. I often came off as pretty spazzy, in fact. For me, the way to *seem* confident, was to *be* confident – which is why I have all these suggestions for being prepared.

If you are one of those gifted beings who simply has *savoir faire*, knows what to do, seems at perfect ease, and will take to the wards like a duck to water, well then: Bully for you! This guide is for the rest of us.

PUNCTUALITY

An easy way to look professional. It's important. 'Nuf said.

SPIN CONTROL: A BALM FOR WHEN YOU BOMB

You will have days when you screw up. Sometimes, only you will notice; other times, you will be made explicitly aware that your teammates have noticed as well.

We all want to do well on the wards. It's possible that, for some of us, even a slight screw-up will make us feel like utter failures. It's important to keep a sense of humor and **keep things in perspective.** Below are a few "war stories" that you can think about the next time you feel like a complete bonehead.

When I was on my medicine clerkship, the program director would have the medical students tour around to each others' patients and demonstrate interesting physical findings. Now, as if I weren't nervous enough about my exam skills, every time I laid hands on a patient, my program director would tell me I was doing the exam wrong. EVERY TIME. Cardiac auscultation, spleen palpation, lung percussion: You name it, I did it wrong. I was sure, since all my evaluations went through this guy, that I was doomed to get a lousy score. The fact that I wanted to go into internal medicine only made me feel worse. Guess what? *I got honors on that rotation.*

Another story: During one of my rotations, I overslept several times during call, arriving late to pre-rounds and often not being able to do even a minimal job of collecting data on my patient. One morning, one of my senior residents approached me afterward, shook her finger in my face, and growled: "I have a bone to pick with you." She then let me know that pre-rounding in 2 minutes was NOT acceptable performance. At the time, I wished the ground would open and swallow me. She was right; I felt terrible. The fact that this had happened more than once made me feel even worse. "Well, I guess I can kiss honors on this rotation good-bye," I thought to myself. Guess what? *I got honors on that rotation, too*. And I'm on very friendly terms with that resident.

A final story: During a stint in the clinics, I assessed a lady with the chief complaint of vertigo. When I presented to my attending, I told him I suspected she was having a stroke. After seeing the patient with me, he came up with a simpler explanation for her dizziness: An ear infection. (All together now: *Oooof!*) Boy, did I feel stupid. And yet, only 20 minutes later, that same attending gave me my end-of-rotation feedback: *He was recommending me for honors.*

The point of these stories is to remind you that one, or a few, mistakes, no matter how excruciating they may feel to you, do not necessarily determine your entire clerkship grade. Your grades are a reflection of total effort over several weeks under many different evaluators. So **don't get overly discouraged** by your screw-ups.

In fact, I would advise, based on the experiences of others, that you be careful not to let your reaction to a mistake lead to so much anxiety that you overcompensate. One friend was so eager to demonstrate an excellent fund of knowledge, in the face of early feedback that his fund was not so good, that he became, in his own judgment, "too pushy" to show his knowledge. This rubbed his teammates the wrong way, leading – as most such "emotional intelligence" factors do – to a global effect on his evaluation. In this case, negative.

At some point after an error (during a break, at home, in the shower . . .), pause, take a breath, and think about how you will do things differently from now on to avoid repeating the mistake. It sucks to screw up, but it sucks worse if you don't improve from your mistakes. So analyze them.

GUNNERS: THE DEMON WITHIN

What's a gunner? Some people define it as "an ambitious person focused on getting a great evaluation." I do not think that's a gunner; I think that describes most of us in medical school. I would define a gunner as "an ambitious person focused on getting a great evaluation ... *to the detriment of others, including his patients or his peers.*"

Many of my classmates have complained to me of gunner behavior by peers on the wards that they found annoying, disturbing, aggravating, and unfair. And I think it's true that when we think of the "problem" of "gunning," we usually think of it in terms of other people's behavior.

I would suggest, however, that the problem of gunning begins at home. In other words: **Beware the gunner within.** How to do this? It's inevitable, after about the first week of clerkships, that you will notice that some of your peers are going to be doing excellent work. And, in the new era of being evaluated, one's conditioning might lead one to feel insecure, and even jealous, of that person's good standing with the team. If you notice yourself developing such feeling about a classmate, stop yourself. Instead of indulging your inner child's whining, "Why don't they give gold stars to ME?" ask yourself, "**What is this person doing that I can emulate?**" If you have a peer who seems to have what it takes to perform well on the wards, STUDY THEM. They've obviously figured out what works.

To indulge the jealous or competitive impulse, on the other hand, leads to very bad behavior – even if we're not the ones perpetrating it. As one example, on one of my clerkships, I noticed that one of my peers got into the habit of correcting things I said in front of my residents. Now, sometimes he was right, but I noticed that he was also doing it even when he was incorrect. Apparently he thought correcting my "errors" (even when I didn't make any) made him look smarter. And my confidence was so shaken, I actually started to believe he was right about things, even when he got it wrong. When it reached that point, I resolved to speak to him in private about it, gently draw his attention to what he was doing (since I was *sure* [wink-wink] he wasn't doing this on *purpose*), and ask him not to do it.

As a general guideline for all medical students, might I suggest the following: **Show your peers the courtesy of never correcting**

them in front of their evaluators, unless it poses an immediate health risk to a patient. You can gently correct them behind the scenes, if you must. If a public correction is needed, let it be done by the resident or attending – not by you.

Many students complain about peer behaviors that are not exactly wrong, but seem phony or unfair, such as kissing up, making small talk with attendings about their personal interests, using personal connections to socialize with superiors outside of the wards, or even flirting with superiors. Students complain that people engaging in such behaviors may have crummy patient skills or lousy funds of knowledge, but thanks to such "butt-kissing" they are still able to do well.

Let's use some of the advice from our discussion to dissect these complaints. First of all, your concern should be with your own conduct and performance. If *you're* doing an excellent job, what *they* do shouldn't matter as much. As far as such behavior giving an unfair advantage, I agree flirting is simply unethical, and I would not engage in it. As for using personal connections, that's something you either have or you don't. Some people are born looking like movie stars, and the rest of us aren't, and that doesn't seem fair either, but that's life. In the long run, relying on such behaviors to advance is a crutch that weakens a person's reliance on their own internal resources. Such a person is destined for eventual trouble. Not recommended.

But what about "**butt-kissing**"? Here's a weird idea: What if some of those behaviors were not seen as butt-kissing, but rather as a form of "schmoozing," or professional networking? Rather than sullenly focusing our jealousy at the unfair advantage such behaviors give our "competitors," consider whether such behaviors are actually genuinely friendly and an attempt to make a connection with someone. In other words, maybe your peer is exhibiting a form of emotional intelligence in strengthening their rapport with a member of the team. Their ability to do this may be unique to them, but it might also be a skill you can study and learn from. While **I don't suggest you do anything that would** feel **"phony"** or "fake" or "cheesy," I think you should consider finding ways in which you, too, might make a personal connection with teammates.

Perhaps part of why butt-kissing bothers us is that we feel the butt-kissers do it so they can slack off on other parts of their work and still get a good evaluation. In other words, we suspect they're lazy. We might also feel that these people are only looking out for their own well-being, and not for their patients' or anyone else's. In other words, they're gunners, in my use of the word.

We don't have any control over other people's motivations. But I would say, **if your heart and motivation are in the right place, there's no harm in borrowing the tactics of the butt-kissers** to accomplish your own, hopefully more meritable, goals.

* * *

SECTION X

Team Management for the MS3

Here are a few suggestions for helping you in dealing with team dynamics.

LOGISTICS

First of all, make sure you introduce yourself to ALL team members; not just docs but also NPs, pharmacists, social workers, translators, etc. – anyone who rounds with your group. Every team member is a potential ally who may help you. So be friendly, **know everyone's name, and use it.** This also applies to nurses staffing wards your patients are on.

Also, have a card for recording your R1, R2/3, and attendings' pager numbers. I also make a point of noting down my residents' institutional physician code number, as well as licence number and DEA number for attendings. These codes are needed on order forms for labs and studies, and I usually have an opportunity to collect them during the course of work in the first week or two and jot them down where I keep pager numbers. Residents and attendings like it when you fill out forms for their sign-off with the codes already filled in; it shows you're paying attention.

In most cases, students are allowed to write orders, as long as they're cosigned by an intern or resident. Talk to your team about how they want to manage this. Also, as noted elsewhere in this volume, medication orders should ALWAYS be double-checked against a reference manual. Medication errors are a common cause of bad events.

GREAT EXPECTATIONS: SOLICITING FEEDBACK

Make it a habit, soon after joining a team, to speak to your evaluators. (Those are usually your attending and senior resident, and not your interns, but this varies, so check with your program director.) Let them know what your personal goals are for the rotation, and find out what their expectations are for you. Also, during the first conversation, tentatively suggest picking a date, about halfway into the rotation, when you would like to meet with them to discuss how you're doing on the clerkship. On busy services, they may not want to set a time and simply ask you to come find them when the time arrives.

Initiating this conversation demonstrates a high degree of professionalism, which, as explained, helps you in areas you wouldn't even expect.

GAUGING YOUR TEAM; OR, KNOW WHEN TO TREAD LIGHTLY

Unfortunately, skills such as being able to accurately read when your resident is too tired to answer questions, or whether an attending is rather formal or someone who appreciates a good joke, is not something that can be imparted with advice. I'm not even sure if it can be taught. But I can tell you that people who can read their team members in this way – that is, who demonstrate "emotional intelligence" – are going to fare better than those who cannot.

"YES, VIRGINIA, THERE IS SUCH A THING AS A STUPID QUESTION"

Related to the above, but more substantive: While in lecture we were assured constantly that there are no dumb questions, this is not necessarily true on the wards. Specifically, I make it a policy

never to ask questions about basic information I could glean from a textbook. Why annoy your superiors with such questions when you can educate yourself on the issue – and maybe learn some things your attending had forgotten? (And by the way, if you ask such questions, you will likely be told, "Good question. Why don't you look it up and let us know tomorrow?")

When I ask questions, I try to **make them about the resident's clinical judgement** – something I can't learn from a book – **or about my patient's particular case.** Examples: Not "What kind of murmur do you hear in a patient with mitral stenosis?" but rather, "What do you find works the best to elicit the murmur when you examine a patient with mitral stenosis?" Not "What drugs will we use for Mrs. Gonzalez's myocardial infarction?" but rather, "How will Mrs. Gonzalez's renal failure affect our choice of drugs for her myocardial infarction?"

While asking questions can be a way to demonstrate interest in your patients' problems, BE CAREFUL to follow this advice. I had one friend who, while sitting around with her resident on call, asked a lot of basic questions about anti-arrhythmics – a topic that, frankly, even most attendings find a little complicated. My friend thought she was demonstrating an interest in her patient. Her resident, instead, cited the conversation in his evaluation as evidence of her "poor fund of knowledge." (All together now: *Oooof!*) The lesson: Never ask basic questions of a superior when you can check a book. In fact, by reading up, you may be able to ask smarter questions and come off as more informed than your intern!

THE REST OF THE TEAM: TIPS TO WORKING WITH OTHER STAFF

Most students have some sense of the members of the physician team (attending, senior resident, intern, subintern, clerk, or MS3), but keep in mind that you will be working with many members of other health professions on your teams, in the clinics and on the wards. Some of them could be crucial allies.

Nurses. The first commandment of clerkships: **Nurses can be the medical student's best friend.** I think it's wise to befriend the NPs on your team, if there are any. They are usually the best teachers, especially in physical exam skills, and are often friendlier than the doctors. Ward RNs can also be very helpful in keeping you informed about your patient – so make it a point to meet them and communicate with them regularly. Ward nurses spend more time with your patient than you do and may notice things you do not.

Social workers. Again, these folks are important to know about. Especially if you have a patient with "dispo" issues – homeless, frail elderly, psych issues – the social worker is key to finding a safe and efficient discharge plan. On some services, in fact, teams have social workers or nurses whose only job is to ensure secure discharges for the patients.

Rehabilitation services, or PT/OT/ST. To the detriment of our patients, the therapists, and ourselves, *housestaff have a PROFOUND ignorance of the skills and function of rehab therapists.* This section gives you more and better-organized information about PT/OT/ST than I was able to pick up on my own during three years on the wards. I kept waiting for a formal introduction to this topic, and I never got it. If you read this section, it will put you ahead of many interns and residents.

Many housestaff (and even attendings!) give a rehab services consultation about as much thought as blowing their noses. Frequently they meld PT and OT together, as if they were one service (they're absolutely distinct), as in, "This patient's looking sort of sluggish. Call PT/OT and have them see her." All too often R1s give an urgent call to PT on discharge day to "bless" the patient before she's shuffled out the door – which treats PT's assessment as little more than a pro forma duty. In many cases it's not needed at all, but if you really think PT is needed, don't call at the last minute, unless you're arranging home PT services for the patient after discharge.

BEFORE YOU CALL REHAB, you should:

(1) find out something about the patient's baseline function. For example, did he use a cane or walker at home? (Don't assume he didn't just because he didn't have it when he arrived at the hospital – patients usually leave them at home.) Family or friends can be helpful in fleshing this out.

(2) Once you know the baseline function, ask yourself: Is the patient at their baseline now, or do you feel they've lost ground since being admitted to the hospital, either due to their illness or just deconditioning from sitting around? **If you aren't sure the patient is at his or her baseline, or you feel their functional status could be better than it is now, AND the patient is physically and mentally ready to work with a therapist, call rehab services.** Don't order rehab for patients who are at their baseline; this includes patients with significant but stable deficits – e.g., a quadriplegic who is stably at his baseline level of function. For obvious reasons, don't order rehab for a patient in the throes of alcohol withdrawal.

(3) Make sure, if necessary, you have changed the patient's "activity" order from "bedrest" or "non-weight-bearing" to a status compatible with rehab activity, i.e., "mobilize as tolerated" or whatever your resident/intern deems appropriate. Make sure other services are contacted if pertinent; e.g., discuss activity levels with ortho service if the patient is post-op and ortho is following the case.

(4) Identify which rehab therapist is going to be most helpful:

- *Physical therapists* assess patients' gross motor skills, such as how they're walking and if they're at risk of falling. Consult PT for gait training, functional mobility training, assessing a patient's need for a cane or walker, and range of motion exercising for ICU patients.
- *Occupational therapists* assess more fine motor, activity of daily living[1] (ADL) type skills, such as being able to cook a meal,

---

[1] ADLs = feeding, bathing, hygiene, dressing, toilet and tub transfers on own.

groom, etc. They also take care of upper extremity splinting, hand rehab, assessment of general cognitive function and problem solving, and range of motion exercises for ICU patients (as PT does).

- *Speech therapists* not only analyze problems with speech production but may also be able to assess whether a patient is at risk of choking or has "airway issues," which they can do with a swallow study, including a modified barium swallow study if needed.

Make sure your consult form includes complete information about previous baseline function and specific questions/goals for the consult therapist. And again, don't consult on the day of discharge.

And finally: Some teams consult rehab to assess a patient's suitability to go to a rehab facility, or "rehab SNF"[2] (see Appendix 2, "Dispo Dancing," for more on this). Patients need to be strong enough to tolerate three hours a day of exercise to be eligible for rehab SNF. Otherwise, they can go to a regular SNF. If a patient is going to go to a SNF anyway and is NOT in need of rehab (i.e., fully functional patient needing IV antibiotics), don't consult PT/OT "for SNF." It's a waste of time.[3]

PATIENT CARE: THEIR CATS WILL THANK YOU

Students often feel uncertain about their role on the doctor team. I think it's important to remember that students have more time with the patients than do residents or attendings. Thus, you are the "fingers" of the team – **you are the "human touch" in patients' medical care.** Don't forget this, and don't think that just because you don't see residents spending time chatting with patients, that you shouldn't do this. Good residents will explain to you that even though *they* don't have time to do those things, they support your doing them and even expect you to do them.

---

[2] SNF = skilled nursing facility – i.e., a nursing home.
[3] Tips on working with rehab therapists are taken from handout by the San Francisco General Hospital Rehabilitation Department.

One of my patients, a lady with mesenteric ischemia, had post-surgery complications and wound up in the CCU. She had no family or friends nearby, and, being on a ventilator, couldn't talk. She had been a journalist before retirement, as I had been before med school, and we bonded about both being writers. Anyway, the evening after she woke up in the CCU, I stopped by to read to her (Walt Whitman, to be exact). The sight of a "whitecoat" reading to his patient was apparently surprising – the visiting nurse actually asked me if I was her relative! "I'm just her medical student," I explained. I may have felt a little awkward, but it meant something to her, and I'm glad I did it, because she never left that hospital.

Another one of my patients, a lady with pneumonia, was very anxious to leave the hospital. When I probed a little, she told me she had three cats at home and no one to feed them. So, I borrowed her keys, stopped by the house, and fed the cats. My residents all chuckled about this, but hey – who else was gonna feed her cats? If my mom was in the hospital with no one to feed her pets, I'd hope some nice medical student would do that for her.

Do these things. They matter. And students can do them better than the rest of the team.

COMMUNICATON: BE LIKE ERNESTINE[4]

One very important role you can play in patient care is enhancing communication. Like a telephone switchboard operator, you are the interface between the care team and the patient. I have two main points about team-related communiqués with patients: (1) orientation of your patient to the team-based academic medical system and (2) translation of "Doctorese."

Many patients hospitalized for the first time (or the fourth, or eighth . . .) don't understand the hierarchy of an academic medical

[4] Ernestine the Operator is a famous character played by Lily Tomlin on the 1960s show *Laugh-In*. She was more often known for her mis-communication skills, so perhaps I should exhort you to be *better* than Ernestine, but she was also charming and down-to-earth, as any good medical student ought to be.

center, are baffled by the seemingly endless parade of whitecoats, and can't keep tabs on who's who among their care team. In fact, I heard a story of a patient who told the team attending that the medical student was his doctor: "I don't know who the rest of you interlopers are!"

When I introduced myself to a patient, I explained that I was a medical student – a "junior doctor-in-training." I also explained that the intern was my "boss," and that the resident was *her* boss, and that our attending was the *resident's* boss. I explained that doctors often traveled in packs, "like wolves," with the attending being the "alpha wolf" with the most experience and the ultimate responsibility. I also explained that, although the attending was in charge, it was the *resident* who spent the most time, day in and day out, in the hospital. A special "night doctor" (nightfloat) was available to take care of problems on nights when the team was at home. Finally, I explained that in addition to the main team, the patient might see other specialty "consulting" teams or "packs" – e.g., infectious disease, GI – while in hospital.

"I don't wanna be a guinea pig." Most patients, if they think of the hierarchy at all, express concern that they not be "guinea pigs" with inexperienced persons practicing on them for procedures. Patients may not, however, understand who has the most experience. Certainly for a surgery, the attending has the most experience and would be present during an operation; you may mention that your role, if any, might be to simply watch the operation or hold a retractor. On the other hand, for ward procedures such as a lumbar tap or central line, the resident often is more in practice than the attending. (I recall one patient insisting that the attending, being the "alpha wolf," do his tap – not realizing that this particular attending hadn't done one in years! *"Um, sir, you might want to reconsider . . . "*)

You should explain to patients that at an academic medical center, **the junior doctors learn by doing procedures WITH the senior doctors,** *together.* That said, you should reassure them that the *team* works for *them*, and if they are uncomfortable with a planned procedure, they are always free to refuse it or request someone else to do it.

In addition to preparing the patient for team-based care, you should **warn them that communication among all the doctors is NOT INSTANTANEOUS,** and that the patient may be told one thing by one team or doctor in the morning and be told something totally different an hour later. This is simply a function of "who gets the news first," and patients may need to bear with the team as information percolates across teams and down the line of command. Such a warning can prevent needless confusion and even anger on the part of the patient. And it's easy for you to do.

Translation of Doctorese. I have often been astonished at what *very basic* information patients do not receive – or perhaps do not comprehend – during hospitalization. Patients may not understand the planned treatment, the chance of success, even their diagnosis – or at least the list of possible diagnoses.[5]

Recently, as an attending, I admitted a patient to the hospital. On the planned day of discharge, I received a note in clinic from the client informing me that he was not going home. When I called him, I asked him why he wasn't being discharged, and he replied, "I have no idea. The day they pulled my PICC,[6] they took a picture of it, and then the doctor came in and said I had to stay three more days, and they gave me shots in the stomach." It took me a couple of seconds to realize the patient had developed a venous thrombus – a common complication in patients with central lines, treated with enoxaparin injections. It is possible that the resident explained this to the client, but because it was given in "Doctorese," or technical jargon, he understood very little of it.

---

[5] I have noticed that some patients with no evidence of cognitive dysfunction may need to be told many times that they have cancer – it's as if their brain has difficulty holding such painful information.

[6] Peripheral intravenous central catheter – i.e., a large IV "central line" that is inserted through a vein in an extremity rather than the usual femoral, jugular, or subclavian sites. PICCs are more durable and suited to patients who need weeks of IV treatment – e.g., antibiotics for endocarditis or osteomyelitis.

Although we may believe we doctors still speak in English, in point of fact we learn a very different language that is confusing to laypersons, especially those with hearing deficits or for whom English is not the primary language. **As the medical student, you are still learning this jargon, and so you speak a type of "pidgin English"** that may still be comprehensible to the average sick layperson. Translating complicated medical concepts into plain English can be tough, especially when you do not understand all the technical details yourself, but patients are often satisfied with at least the same level of understanding, in lay terms, that you have as their medical student. Thus, it is never wrong to frequently ask your patient, "Do you understand why we think you are sick? Do you understand what we plan to do to treat you? Do you have questions?" You'll often be surprised at the wildly cockeyed misapprehensions they have of what's going on with their bodies, illness, and care plans. You have a great opportunity to allay fears and clarify misconceptions – which greatly improves outcomes. (Ignorant patients, for example, are much more likely to fail to adhere to treatment when they leave the hospital, increasing the risk of a bounce-back and continued illness or death.)

That said, **if you have a major question** yourself about the case – e.g., exactly what happens in the surgery, or the long-term prognosis of the likely diagnosis, or whether to tell the patient that cancer is a leading explanation for their symptoms – **talk to your seniors about it before discussing with the patient.** You don't want to give the patient a wrong explanation or disclose information that your senior would rather not disseminate yet.

* * *

SECTION XI

Morale Management

There are three elements: time, your mental/emotional health, and your physical health.

TIME MANAGEMENT: THE CRUCIAL SURVIVAL SKILL

At my orientation, a UCSF faculty member, Dr. Ellen Hughes, told a horror story about being advised before her clerkships to buy 30 pairs of underwear, because she wouldn't have time to wash them!

I was relieved to find that I had time to wash my underwear. And even my socks. Even during inpatient rotations, you will **usually have your weekends off.** My advice: USE THEM. Use your weekends to at least do your laundry and buy food for the week. I also adopted a "same day" policy on paying my bills – in other words, as soon as I opened it I wrote a check and dropped it in the mail.

Doing chores like this, especially when you're tired, is a pain. But it keeps the work week saner. **It may suck to spend part of Saturday at Costco, but it sucks more to get home at 8:00 P.M. after a long day and have nothing to eat.**

If you're already on top of stuff like this, breathe easy – you will probably be able to maintain that. If you're not, getting more organized will help you to stay sane.

Also, many people post-call have an adrenaline surge going and may be tempted to go out with friends, etc. after work. This may be an act of resistance, fighting the feeling that med school is "stealing" your life away. I STRONGLY RECOMMEND the following activity, post-call: sleep. If you don't, it'll catch up with you. **Your cosmetologist will thank you later.**

MENTAL AND EMOTIONAL PREPARATION

You may be entering third year feeling pretty good, pretty confident, pretty together. Or you may be feeling very anxious. Either way, it's wise to prepare for emotional turbulence ahead. It's better to plan for needing extra support, and find you don't need it, than to go in thinking you'll be fine, and then **finding out the hard way that thanks to unnoticed depression or stress, you've been a grouch** and alienated people around you – including your evaluators.

Marshal support. There are various ways to do this. In my case, my partner was more proactive in "battening down the hatches" in preparation for third year than I was. He helped me get my clothes and gear together, and for the first few weeks he packed lunches for me. (I know, I know, if I weren't already married to him, this would be a reason to do so.)

If you have a partner, I *don't* necessarily suggest you find a way to get him or her to make you lunches, but you might give a warning that the months ahead will be stressful and that understanding and support will be especially important to you.

And, regardless of whether you're single or in a relationship, you should **warn your family** and non-school friends that you are entering a stressful period and will need extra support. If they want to see you, maybe they should drive to your place – you might be too tired to travel to see them. Heck, they might even take you out to dinner. (Well, it can't hurt to ask; show them this guide and tell them it'll get you into AOA.) Likewise, they shouldn't expect that you will be instantly reachable by phone.

The **non-school sources of support become especially important** since you're unlikely to see your classmates much, and when you talk to them, they may be as stressed out and tired as you are. On the other hand, many students mention that third year gave them a chance to bond with classmates they barely knew during the first two years, who became good friends. Still. . . .

Third year can be isolating. Many students are surprised to find they feel isolated in third year, despite being surrounded by people all day long. You don't see your class pals on a daily basis anymore, unless they're randomized to your clerkship site with you. And even though you'll have residents around you on your "team," you may feel obligated to keep your "stage face" and not let loose about how stressed out you are. In fact, they may be the very people about whom you need to vent!

Many medical schools have **student support groups** or **well-being programs.** Make sure that you are at least aware of such programs at your institution and take advantage of them if need be. Many students find having a place to vent during the first months of clerkship is very helpful.

In my own case, I prepared for the emotional stresses of third year by visiting student health services. I told the psychiatrist about my history of depression and my worries that clerkship stresses might get me down. She took a full history from me and we planned for me to watch my moods and to come back if it felt like I was getting depressed so that I could discuss treatments, including antidepressants. She assured me that my medical records at SHS were completely confidential. As it turned out, I was able to manage my moods fine, but it felt good to have a backup plan.

PHYSICAL PREPARATION

(Cue *Rocky* theme song.) Regular exercise is possible during third year – you may not be able to go to the gym three times a week, but even on surgery I was able to go one or two times a week. If you like going to the gym, you should be able to keep doing it, although sometimes not as often. If you're a couch potato: That's a problem, and I'm putting you on notice, right now, that **you need to get**

regular exercise. A sedentary lifestyle will lead to worse health later. If you're serious about working in health care, you need to lead by example. There's no excuse for health care providers not to be engaged in regular exercise, even if it's only walking for 30 minutes a day. So do it.

Food. Obviously, this varies by institution, but as a general rule, if you rely on getting it from your workplaces, **you're going to be eating a lot of bad, and often expensive, food.** I didn't think it was possible to find food worse than SF General's cafeteria, until I went to the San Francisco VA. *Oooo-weee!*

Some clerkships will give you accounts for free or discounted meals at the cafeterias. Usually your dinner on-call will be free. This may make it worthwhile to obtain food from the hospital. Also, many departments provide free pizza, burritos, or the like for noontime lectures – food paid for by drug companies. It's not the healthiest stuff, and some of you may have reservations about eating on a drug company's tab.[1] I suggest bringing lunches whenever possible – they'll be healthier and probably more appetizing, but packing them will take time.

---

[1] Comment: The June 22, 2000, *New England Journal of Medicine* featured an excellent, and overdue, editorial about the abuses by the U.S. drug industry. It may seem that buying lunch for a bunch of tired, overworked students and residents is harmless. But companies have the excess money to throw around on such perks for us because of their de facto monopolies and exploitation of U.S. consumers, who pay for companies' huge profit margins. Such perks have been shown to influence prescribing practices. I'm not trying to rain on the parade; in third year I did at times indulge in a free lunch (but usually I packed my own). Still, it's important to remember that **there's no such thing as a truly free lunch.** Medical students and doctors can take an individual pledge to decline drug company promotions – including the often slanted promotional literature handed out during lunch – at **www.nofreelunch.org**.

* * *

SECTION XII

Soapbox: Physicians and the Snare of Egoism

Physicians are notoriously self-involved. This country's traditional medical culture reinforces narcissism and competitiveness in its members, almost from the first day of pre-medical training. While being concerned for one's own personal well-being is a natural human trait, when taken to extremes it can produce a great deal of disharmony. In the case of our own profession, overemphasis on the physician as the center of her own universe has led to some of the unnecessarily brutal aspects of medical training in this country. It also explains why our profession, more than any other allied health profession, is struggling enormously in the face of a changing American health care system.

Many doctors in this country still operate as if it's 1970-something, and each doctor is his own corporation: "I am Dr. Bob Jones, Inc." At most, they might conceive of themselves as part of a small group of affiliated fellow physicians. This fails to face up to reality: To managed care and to integrated health systems, **we are widgets** – cogs in their machines. The fact that I, Dr. Bob Jones, am especially skilled in taking care of older patients, or catching tricky diagnoses, or working with depressed patients, or whatever – whatever individual skills I've cultivated in myself in which I take great pride – is totally invisible to the health care corporations.

American doctors persist in the delusion of themselves as individual corporate entities. Their interest in maintaining their individuality, self-determination, and mild competitiveness against their peers, above and beyond any inclination to cooperate with those peers, is part of why doctors are failing so miserably to adapt to the rapid changes in U.S. health economics. If you could give out letter grades to the health professions for adjusting to the new conditions, doctors would get an *L* – for *Losers*. Our inadequacy is especially clear when you compare us to nurses, PAs, PTs – most of the other professions are thriving. Meanwhile, docs are working harder than ever, yet **satisfaction levels among young primary care doctors are actually *lower* than those for older docs.** I think our profession could get a clue from other professions, such as nurses, in which individuals are unified and cooperate within professional organizations and unions. To thrive, and not just survive, physicians are going to have to start thinking about the well-being of their profession, not just of their own specialty or individual practice.

In medical education, the profession has fostered this sense of competition with practices such as numeric rank of students by test performance – as if we were *Fortune* 500 companies whose worth is measured unidimensionally. The unfortunate psychological effects of the ruthless competitiveness fostered by such practices were only slowly realized. There is a reason grades were eliminated at UCSF for the first two years. Some of us wonder what effect it might have to eliminate them from the entire process.

What does this have to do with us? As you embark on the wards, consider how the sense of competitiveness emerges, in yourself and your peers. Resist the temptation to focus on your own performance, to the exclusion or even detriment of your classmates. And consider how an overemphasis on self-interest within our profession as a whole has been our undoing. **If you're going to compete with anyone, compete with yourself.**

Many of us arrive at medical school with the goal of producing one excellent doctor – ourselves. The truth, however, is that **we are here to produce as many excellent doctors as we can** – ourselves, our classmates, our teachers, our residents, and even our attendings. The flow of knowledge on the physician team is not unilateral. We, too, have something to teach our superiors.

I took the effort to assemble these guidelines because I want each and every one of you to be the best you can be on the wards. If these notes have helped you, think about that, and look for opportunities to extend similar assistance to your peers as you wend your way through third year.

I'm sure you'll take good care of your patients on the wards. Take good care of each other, too.

* * *

Tasty Bits: Good Things to Know Up Front

TIPS ON PHARMACOLOGY

You don't have to know the dose and schedule of every drug in the PDR to seem well-informed about drug topics on the wards and clinics. Especially on inpatient wards, a relatively small set of drugs are used over and over, and you would do well to make yourself especially familiar with them. They are anticoagulants (warfarin, heparin, enoxaparin), pain meds (especially opiates), insulin, and bowel regimens (docusate, bisacodyl, Sennokot, and the like).

Bowel drugs. We didn't study them much in pharmacology, but they are handed out like candy on the wards. (For a decent overview, see Prather CM. Evaluation and treatment of constipation and fecal impaction in adults. *Mayo Clin Proc.* 1998;73:881– 887.). Key point: **If you write a scrip for opiates, your next act should be writing scrips for a bowel regimen.** Anyone on opiates should have a standing order for the stool softener docusate (250 mg po bid, hold for loose stools), and a PRN order for a cathartic, either senna tabs (2 tabs po q12h PRN constipation) or bisacodyl. By the way, docusate alone is insufficient for opiate patients, since the problem is decreased peristalsis.

Bowel regimens are serious business. I had a patient who became obstipated despite aggressive management, including enemas, and wound up perforating her colon. She went into hypovolemic shock and almost died. Very, very bad. So treat this issue seriously.

Sliding scale insulin (SSI). This is an example of how insulin orders are commonly written on the wards:

- FSBS q4hrs
- Insulin, regular, human. Sliding scale, given SQ following FSBS[1] level: 0–80, give juice and call HO[2]; 81–200 = 0 units; 201–250 = 4 units; 251–300 = 6 units; 301–350 = 8 units; 351–400 = 10 units; >400, give 12 units and call HO

I did not have any formal reading on "sliding scale insulin" in pharmacology. There's a reason. It's not evidence-based medicine, but it's been around for decades. SSI regimens have the defect of giving insulin *after* high blood sugar levels appear, and not giving any when sugars are normal even if the patient is taking in food destined to raise them. Patients also have to get stuck round-the-clock, even in the middle of the night when they're not eating. SSI is used mainly because it's simple and convenient for housestaff.

Several studies on SSI demonstrate its problems. In one, patients on proactive insulin regimens stayed in the hospital for less time and had lower sugar levels than did SSI patients.[3] In another study, patients on SSI had a three-fold higher risk of hyperglycemia compared to patients on no drug regimen at all![4] For more information on the efficacy of SSI and other "medical myths," see Paauw DS. Did we learn evidence-based medicine in medical school? Some common medical mythology. *JABFP*.1999;12:143–149.

---

[1] Fingerstick blood sugar.

[2] House officer, i.e., intern or resident.

[3] Gearhart JG, et al. Efficacy of sliding-scale insulin therapy: a comparison with prospective regimens. *Fam Pract Res J.* 1994;14:313–322.

[4] Queale WS, et al. Glycemic control and sliding scale insulin use in medical inpatients with diabetes mellitus. *Arch Intern Med.* 1997;157:545–552.

Other sliding scales. Many references, including *The Hospitalist Handbook*, which is available online, include sections with common sliding scales for heparin, K, and Mg.

Pain medication dose conversions. Often you will need to convert one form of pain medication to another, e.g., IV to po, or morphine to fentanyl. The following table, taken from the UCSF Adult Pain Management Guide, should help:

Opioid Analgesic	Equi-analgesic Doses (mg)	
Generic name (Brands)	Oral	Parenteral (IV)
Morphine (Roxanol, MS Contin)	30 mg	10 mg
Hydromorphone (Dilaudid)	7.5 mg	1.5 mg
Oxycodone (Percocet, Oxycontin)	20 mg	–
Methadone (titrate slowly – long half-life)	20 mg (acute)	10 mg (acute)
	2–4 mg (chronic)	2–4 mg (chronic)
Hydrocodone (Vicodin, Lortab, Norco)	30 mg	–
Codeine (Tyco #2 = 15 mg, #3 = 30 mg, #4 = 60 mg)	180–200 mg	130 mg
Fentanyl	–	0.1 mg (100 μg)
Fentanyl transdermal (Duragesic)*	2:1 rule**	–

* The onset of the analgesia is delayed 8–12 hours with fentanyl patch, so other pain medications should continue for the first 12 hours. There is a residual effect even after the patch is removed. Do not use the patch on patients naive to opioids – use other forms to safely titrate them first, then calculate a conversion. Use only in stable chronic pain.

** If the total 24-hour dose of oral morphine is 100 mg, the approximate equi-analgesic dose of transdermal fentanyl is 50 μg/hr or 2:1 equivalency.

Corticosteroids. Steroids are a common class of medications encountered on the wards that, like insulin, have been around long enough that their use is more dictated by tradition than by evidence. Some tips include the following.

Cortisol replacement: Keep in mind that the natural pattern of cortisol secretion causes the highest blood levels in the morning. Previously, patients with adrenal insufficiency were often given hydrocortisone in a schedule of 20 mg of hydrocortisone in the morning and 10 mg in the evening. This, however, does not actually succeed in mimicking natural hormonal patterns because of how hydrocortisone is absorbed. Prednisone 5 mg po qhs is a perfectly acceptable regimen.[5]

"Stress-dose steroids:" Patients who take steroids regularly need stress-dose coverage in the setting of acute illness. A "generic" dose for moderate illness is hydrocortisone, 50 mg IV q8hrs. The dose might be increased to 100 mg q8hrs for more severe stressors, such as in the case of critical illness or major surgery (with the first dose given before induction of anesthesia), and tapered after the first 24 hours. The following page shows a table of corticosteroid equivalencies.

Side effects: Most patients taking steroids should be on a proton-pump inhibitor to avoid gastritis or ulcers. Elevations in blood sugar levels should be anticipated. Also, for patients on prolonged steroid therapy for months (e.g., for rheumatic disorders), prophylaxes against bone loss (formal exercise program, calcium, with or without a bisphosphonate) and against *Pneumocystis* pneumonia (e.g., trimethoprim-sulfamethoxazole) should be addressed.

---

[5] Nieman LK, Orth DN. Treatment of adrenal insufficiency. UpToDate 12.3, accessed Nov. 14, 2004. Available at: http://patients.uptodate.com/topic.asp?file= endo_hor/3060&title=Adrenal%20insufficiency.

Corticosteroid Equivalencies

Corticosteroid	Approximate Equivalent Dose (mg)	Relative Anti-Inflammatory Potency	Relative Mineralocorticoid Potency	Plasma Half-Life (min)	Biologic Half-Life (hours)
Short-acting					
Cortisone	25	0.8	2	30	8–12
Hydrocortisone	20	1	2	80–118	8–12
Intermediate-acting					
Prednisone	5	4	1	60	18–36
Prednisolone	5	4	1	115–212	18–36
Triamcinolone	4	5	0	200+	18–36
Methylprednisolone	4	5	0	78–188	18–36
Long-acting					
Dexamethasone	0.75	20–30	0	110–210	36–54
Betamethasone	0.6–0.75	20–30	0	300+	36–54

ACID–BASE ALGORITHM

When analyzing an arterial blood gas (ABG) result . . .

1. Look at the pH: acidemic or alkalemic.[6]
2. Is the primary problem metabolic, or respiratory? The $PaCO_2$ will tell you.
3. Is the patient compensating for the problem? Check the HCO_3.
   - If adjusting acutely, the pH changes 0.8 for every 10 of the $PaCO_2$.
   - If patient has had time to adjust, it's 0.3 pH/10 pts $PaCO_2$.
4. Calculate the anion gap: $Na - Cl - HCO_3$ = gap (8–12 = normal, no gap).
   - Low albumin makes gap artificially low; add 2 to the gap for each point of albumin below normal.
   - If gap is >12, patient has a gap acidosis ("MUDPILERS"); >20 is severe.
5. Calculate the "delta gap": the measured gap – 12 = delta gap, also called the "gap-gap."
6. Add the delta gap to the HCO_3:
   - If >30, patient also has a metabolic alkalosis (beyond whatever else is going on);
   - If <23, patient has a metabolic, non-gap acidosis (again, in addition to other issues).

Special note: An anion gap of 12 ("normal") may indicate acidosis in multiple myeloma.

Metabolic gap acidosis: "Mudpilers:" Methanol, uremia, DKA, para-formaldehyde, iron/isoniazid, lactic acidosis, ethanol/ethylene glycol (antifreeze), rhabdomyolysis, salicylates (also later sepsis, which is really lactic acidosis; early sepsis is marked by a respiratory alkalosis).

Metabolic non-gap acidosis: excessive loss of HCO_3: Renal tubular acidosis (RTA), or "Rectal tubular acidosis" – i.e., diarrhea.

---

[6] Not "alkalotic/acidotic," until you determine the process that's producing the pH.

Metabolic alkalosis "HIGH PH:" Hyperaldosteronism (i.e., Conn's), iatrogenic (i.e., diuretics), gastric loss, hypercortisolism (i.e., Cushing's), parathyroidism, hypercalcemia.

- If urine chloride is low: vomiting/NG tube; past diuretic use; post-hypercapnea.
- If urine chloride is normal or high: excess mineralocorticoids (Cushing's, Conn's); current or recent diuretic use; excess alkali administration.

(For more detail, see excellent article by Haber R. A practical approach to acid-based disorders, *West J Med*. 1991;155:146–151.)

APPROACH TO THE CHEST X-RAY

You should be taught how to read chest x-rays on your medicine clerkship. However, you may not get to medicine until the end of the year, and you may get pimped on reading a chest x-ray sometime before then. As with most procedures at this stage of the game, I think most of your superiors will be satisfied if you demonstrate you have a *method* for approaching a task, rather than simply getting the answer.

If someone holds up a CXR film and asks you to read it, I suggest you explain what you're doing as you go. Example: "Well, let's see. The tag indicates this is a film of patient John Smith. It's a chest film . . . looks a little fuzzy, and the heart's a little big, which makes me think it's AP . . . and the tag indicates it's an AP film, anyway, so that confirms it. The inspiration looks like it's down to about rib 10, I can see the spinous processes, clavicles look even, so, good quality film. And . . . I don't see any obvious bone or soft tissue lesions. I see the gastric bubble below the diaphragm, the mediastinum is centered and not enlarged. I see the cardiac borders clearly and the silhouette is not enlarged, and the lung fields appear clear, no densities. Normal chest." By "milestoning" your read, you let your superior see that you have a systematic way of going about it.

The following is a systematic approach to the chest x-ray.

1. **Confirm the name of the patient.**
2. **Evaluate film quality.** The mnemonic is "PIER": position, inspiration, exposure, rotation.
   - **Position:** Typically, upright PA and lateral. Sick patients will have the fuzzier supine AP (because the film is slid under their chest as they are lying down).
   - **Inspiration:** Lung fields should extend to about 10th or 11th rib.
   - **Exposure:** If the film is penetrated enough, you should be able to make out the spinous processes "inside" the vertebrae. If the film is underexposed/too white, you won't be able to see them. If the film is overexposed/too black, bony details will be lost.
   - **Rotation:** Space between the medial clavicle and the margin of the adjacent vertebra should be equal on the right and left sides.
3. **Check the bones:** Scapula, humerus, shoulder joint, clavicle, vertebrae, ribs. Look for lytic lesions, new or old fractures, symmetry, osteoporosis, scoliosis, rib notching.
4. **Check soft tissue:** Breast shadows, supraclavicular regions, axillae, chest wall. Look for thickness, subcutaneous emphysema (air bubbles – dark spots), calcifications (bright spots).
5. **Diaphragm:** Outline should be smooth curves taking off from the midline at 10th–11th rib. Locate gastric air bubble. Look for pneumoperitoneum.
6. **Mediastinum:** Check trachea – should be to right of midline as it approaches carina. Note the great vessels, especially the aortic arch. Look for adenopathy, mass lesions.
7. **Cardiac silhouette:** Check size and shape of heart. Right border should be a finger width to the right of spine. Left border should be distinguishable. Heart width should be less than half of the widest chest diameter.
8. **Lungs:** Check one field, then the other, then compare. Is vasculature engorged? What about the bronchial tree? CP angles

visible? Pneumothorax (check very carefully at the apices)? Pleural thickening? Infiltrates? Cavitation?

- **When describing what you're seeing in the lung fields of a CXR, describe the pattern, but don't diagnose.** Don't say "Looks like fluid in the fields." Say, "<u>I see patchy densities bilaterally</u>, with a silhouette sign obscuring the left cardiac border. <u>This is an alveolar pattern</u> that could be due to pus, such as from pneumonia, or from fluid due to pulmonary edema."

- **Types of lung densities**
  1. **Alveolar:** patchy, poorly marginated. Represents material other than air in the airspaces. May see "air bronchograms" – black lines representing air-filled bronchi amidst water-density alveoli. May note "silhouette signs" – organs' margins blurred by dense material in alveoli of nearby lung tissue.
  2. **Interstitial:** thickening of bronchi, septae. Linear or finely granular patterns of abnormal shadows. "Kerley's B-lines" (not "curly" B-lines) are thickening of interlobular septae and are small, bright, horizontal lines seen especially toward the bases of the lungs. They are associated with CHF. The interstitial pattern is seen in CHF, interstitial fibrosis, cancer, inflammation.
  3. **Atelectasis:** loss of volume → shift of interlobar fissures and mediastinum toward the collapsed region.
  4. **Nodules:** one or more dense, bright, round lesions. Adenoma, granuloma, cancer, cyst, lymph node, etc.
  5. **Other:** abscess (lucency within density, air–fluid level), pneumatoceles (air-containing spaces seen with some pneumonias), honeycombing (airspaces with thick septae).

(The above is adapted from notes by Dr. Hugo Yang, chief resident, Mt. Zion Hospital, San Francisco, autumn 1999, as well as teaching materials from Dr. Marcia McCowan of the Department of Radiology, VAMC, San Francisco.)

APPROACH TO THE ECG

On the wards, no one is going to expect you to diagnose Wolff–Parkinson–White syndrome on your first ECG read. As with the CXR read, they want you to show that you have a *method* for doing the read.

As noted, Dr. Thomas Evans wrote a nifty little set of crib sheets for analyzing ECGs, but his book is a little advanced for novices. However, getting used to the "**Litany of Categorization**," outlined as follows, allows you to eventually take advantage of the Evans method. I first learned this approach from a talk by Dr. Paul Varosy, who is now a cardiologist at UCSF.

Recall the basic shape of the ECG wave (P, QRS, and T waves). Recall that the ECG paper has large boxes, subdivided into five little boxes. Five big boxes is 1.0 second. One big box is 0.2 sec. One little box is 0.04 sec.

As you look at the ECG, focus on a familiar shaped curve (I usually use lead 2) and answer the following questions:

1. ***What's the rate: slow, normal, or fast?*** Usually printed at the top of the ECG printout.
   - You can also count the number of QRS complexes per large box and estimate. Since each box is 0.2 sec, one QRS per box is about 300 beats per minute (bpm). One complex per two boxes is about 150, one complex per three boxes is 100, and so on. The mantra is: 300–150–100–75–60.
   - Any rate under 60 is bradycardia; 60–100 is normal; over 100 is tachycardia.
2. ***Is the QRS complex wide, or narrow?*** In other words, is it over 12 seconds or under?
   - Again, the width of the QRS is often printed at the top of the ECG sheet, or you can inspect it directly (since each "little box" is 0.04 sec, a QRS complex should not be any more than three little boxes).
   - Narrow QRS complexes indicate impulses are traveling through the normal cardiac electrical circuits. Wide QRS

complexes indicate that impulses are traveling through ectopic channels.

3. *Is the rhythm regular, or irregular?* In other words, is the length between R groups (the R–R length) always the same (regular), or does it change?
   - **If it's regular ...**
     1. *Is it a sinus rhythm?* Are there normal, consistently shaped P waves? Is every P wave followed by only one QRS and does each QRS get followed by only one P wave? That tells you if you have "normal sinus rhythm." The P waves should be erect (look like little hills) in lead 2, and "biphasic" (S-shaped) in lead V-1.
   - **If it's irregular** (i.e., if the R–R length changes over time) ...
     1. *Is it predictable, or is it "irregularly irregular"?* Irregularly irregular is usually an indication of atrial fibrillation.
   At this point, you should be able to use the Evans book to identify a set of likely ECG diagnoses (see Evans, p. 34). The rest of the litany, below, is for completeness.

4. *Is the heart's axis deviated?* I'm not going to get into the relationship between heart position and axis, the various leads, and how/why a shift in the heart's position changes the curve shape on various leads. Look in your physiology books and the Evans book if you want the background. Below is a quick way to assess if the axis is right- or left-shifted.
   - Look at the QRS complex in lead I and lead II.
     1. If the complex from I points down, and the complex from II points up, they are pointing toward, or returning to, each other. Returning = right-shifted.
     2. If the complex in I points up, and the complex in II points down, they are pointing away from each other, or leaving each other. Leaving = left-shifted.

5. *Examine the intervals.*
   - Is the PR interval <0.2 sec (one big box)?
     1. PR intervals >0.2 sec = heart block (HB).

   a. Long PR intervals but otherwise normal trace, with no missing QRS complexes → first-degree HB.
   b. Long PR intervals with some missing QRS complexes → second-degree HB.
      • PR intervals progressively lengthen before the missed QRS = second-degree HB, type 1, a.k.a., "Wenckebach" pattern.
      • PR intervals don't change before missed QRS = second-degree HB, type 2.
   c. If P and QRS are completely dissociated, think third-degree/complete HB.
 • QT interval. As a rule, the QT should be $< \frac{1}{2}$ the R-R interval.
6. ***Look for bundle-branch block.***
 • Look at leads V-1 and V-2.
   1. Right BBB is indicated by QRS complexes that show two symmetrical peaks ("Rabbit ears" = right BBB).
   2. Left BBB is indicated by a deep S wave. See the Evans book for more detail.
7. ***Look for signs of ischemia.***
 • T-wave flattening or inversion is usually the first change seen.
 • ST segment depression indicates a subendocardial injury pattern.
 • ST segment elevation ("tombstoning") indicates an infarct...
   1. With Q waves? Can indicate an evolving infarct.
   2. Without Q waves? Indicates acute myocardial injury.

Note that "Q-wave" and "non-Q-wave" MIs are treated differently.

Again, see the Evans book for more explanation and diagrams.

CARDIAC TESTS YOU MAY NOT HAVE HEARD OF

One thing that annoyed me on the wards was references to cardiac diagnostic tests that I had never heard of. You will hear your residents throw around terms like "Patient had a P-thall in October that showed no abnormalities in uptake," or "P-MIBI results consistent with 80% constriction in the LAD." Excuse me? What's a P-MIBI? Or P-thall?

These terms refer to **imaging tests to assess coronary artery disease.** The tests evaluate the flow of blood through heart tissue. To do them, a patient is either put on a treadmill to exercise – a "stress" test – or is given an infusion of a drug to dilate the vessels chemically, which is a "non-stress" test. The latter type of test can be done using the drug dipyridamole (brand name Persantine®) or using adenosine.

Once blood is flowing, you have to measure it. This is done with scintigraphy – i.e., nuclear imaging tests using radioisotopes. The radioisotopes used are **thallous chloride** (Tl-201) or **technetium** (Tc 99m), which has a short half-life that is extended by linking it to **Sestamibi.** Thallium is a potassium analog and is taken up by cells at a rate proportional to the blood flow. Technetium is a calcium analog and, when hooked with Sestamibi, is also taken up at a rate related to flow.

Thus, a "P-MIBI" is a non-stress test that induces vasodilation with dipyridamole and assesses flow using technetium-Sestamibi as the imaging agent. A "P-thall" is similar, but uses thallium as the imaging agent.

In case there are Godzilla-nerds among you for whom the above was not enough information (God help you), see Chou TM, Amidon TM. Evaluating coronary artery disease non-invasively – which test for whom? *West J Med.* 1994;161:173–180.

FLUID BASICS

From day 1, you will be dealing with fluid management decisions in your ward patients. You probably didn't have much practical instruction on fluid management during the first two years. A lot of unfamiliar terms may be thrown around in the first few weeks, which can be intimidating. These notes are intended to give a basic framework and vocabulary.

1. *Types of fluids used:*

Commonly used fluids are **bolded**. Values are milliequivalents per liter (mEq/L).

D_5 refers to 5% dextrose solution. D_5W indicates dextrose in water.

Lactated Ringer's is a maintenance fluid traditionally favored by surgeons. The lactate is quickly converted to HCO_3 by the liver, then converted to CO_2 in the blood. Thus, not a good choice for a patient who's accumulated high levels of CO_2. On medicine, **D_5 $\frac{1}{2}$ NS** is the typical IVF.

By the way, dextrose is not added to IVF for significant nutritional purposes or to prevent muscle breakdown. It's added to keep the Krebs cycle going (to prevent ketoacidosis).

FLUID	Na	Cl	K	HCO_3	Ca	Osm	kCal/L
Crystalloids **Normal saline (NS)**	154	154				292	
D_5NS	154	154				565	200
$\frac{1}{2}$ NS	77	77				146	
D_5 $\frac{1}{2}$ NS	77	77				420	200
D_5 $\frac{1}{4}$ NS	34	34				330	200
D_5W						274	200
D_{10}W						548	400
Lactated ringer's (LR)	130	104	4	28	3	277	
3% NaCl	513	513				960	
Colloids HESPAN	154	154				310	
Plasminate (5% protein)	145	100	.25			310	
25% albumin	130–160	130–160	1.0			310	

Adapted from Fluid and electrolytes. In Lyerly HK, ed. *Handbook of Surgical Intensive Care*, 2nd ed. St. Louis, MO: Moseby;1989:230. With permission from Elsevier.

2. *How to determine which fluid to use, and at what rate:*
  • First, you must decide if the patient is on **maintenance or resuscitation.**
    a. *Maintenance* means replacing fluids lost from normal physiologic functioning.
    b. *Resuscitation* means patient has past or ongoing fluid losses that need to be replaced, e.g., hemorrhage, diarrhea.
  • **Best maintenance fluid for adults:** D_5 $\frac{1}{4}$ NS + 10–20 mEq KCl
    a. Note: D_5 $\frac{1}{2}$ NS is often used, but that gives 185 mEq of excess Na per day; not a big deal if you have a normal heart, but for older folks or cardiac or renal patients, this might be too much Na. Be aware of this.
    b. Note: K is added to fluids to replace losses. Surgeons tend to add K, internists tend not to, because a patient's K can accumulate, and a high K can put them into a fatal dysrhythmia, whereas hypokalemia is less immediately life-threatening. If you're going to include K in the IV fluid, make sure you're checking lytes every day.
  • **The 4–2–1 rule:** The rate of maintenance infusion is calculated in ccs per hour, based on the patient's weight in kg.
    a. The calculation is 4 cc per kg, per hour, for the first 10 kg of weight; 2 cc per kg, per hour, for the next 10 kg, and 1 cc per kg per hour for the rest of the weight.
    b. A short-cut based on the above is "40 plus the weight in kgs." A 70-kg man would need $40 + 70 = 110$ cc/hr of fluid, or $(4 \times 10) + (2 \times 10) + (1 \times 50) = 110$ cc/hr.
  • **Resuscitation fluid:** LR or NS. Note you should not use D_5 up front, because patients under stress could get quite hyperglycemic, thanks to their high stress, high cortisol, and thus, high counter-regulatory activity. They don't need the extra sugar.

A common error in resuscitation is to run fluids too slowly. In a very dehydrated adult, it is acceptable to give a 1- to 2-liter bolus over 30–120 minutes UNLESS the patient has a cardiac history, in which case a slower rate may be prudent. In children, an acceptable bolus would be 10–20 cc/kg. Note: These fluid choices vary depending on the particular clinical scenario.

ADMITTING A PATIENT: MEG'S LIST

On call nights, you will help to admit a patient, including doing your own H&P. I'm not going to go into how to do that – except to reassure you that you *can* do it, and that I strongly recommend Sapira's as a guide for enhancing basic H&P skills. I do have some pre- and post-admission tips.

This may seem obvious, but when your R2 says, "I've got a patient for you," make sure you get the patient's name, date of birth (DOB), and/or medical record number. Your R2 may not have all of this info, but try to get it – it may be important in locating patients who have already been sent up from the ER. If there's time, you will be able to read previous discharge summaries from the patient's computerized medical record, giving you a leg up.

After admission, it's a good idea to review some issues commonly forgotten in the rush of admission, especially in the wee hours. The following checklist is called "Meg's List," and was created by one of my mentors, Dr. Meg Newman. She hands it out to all her teams. You should glance at Meg's List every day when you think about your patients to avoid common management errors. This version of the list was current as of spring 2005.

Meg's List

1. *Precautions*. Some patients may need orders for special sets of standard precautions by nursing staff. The order for these would be "Aspiration precautions" or similar. They include:
   - Aspiration precautions, e.g., past or acute stroke with esophageal dysmotility;
   - Seizure precautions, e.g., alcoholic with past seizure being treated for withdrawal;
   - Fall, e.g., any patient with altered gait;
   - Don't forget prophylaxis for DVT and gastritis or GI bleeding (see "To create an assessment and plan" in Section V for more on this).

2. *Drug interactions and side effects*. Anticipate these before you prescribe every and any medication. Run your patients' meds through a drug interaction program to assess for drug interactions upon admission or before starting any new drug.[7]

3. *Renal dosing*. If this patient has a kidney disorder, new or old, they will likely need lower doses of common meds. Meds needing adjusted dosing for people with kidney disease include, but aren't limited to,

   - *Antibiotics:* acyclovir, aminoglycosides, many antiretrovirals for HIV, most cephalosporins, fluconazole, penicillins, trimethoprim-sulfamethoxazole (e.g., Bactrim®, Septra®), vancomycin.
   - H_2 *blockers:* cimetidine, ranitidine, famotidine.
   - *NSAIDs* – Caution! PGE_2 inhibition can put underperfused kidneys into crisis.
   - *Digoxin*.
   - *Magnesium* in antacids; use with caution.
   - *Enoxaparin:* contraindicated in patients with renal insufficiency.

4. *Ordering antibiotics*. When admitting a sick patient with active infection, make sure to write an order for "STAT" dose, and VERBALLY COMMUNICATE this with the floor nurse when the patient arrives on the floor. Otherwise, the dose will not happen, and in some cases this delay could be very harmful. In some hospitals you must simultaneously fill out a special "antibiotic order sheet" to start the meds. Some hospital pharmacy services automatically shut off empiric antibiotics (i.e.,

---

[7] NB: Meg and I have become fans of the web-based drug interactions algorithm on AIDSmeds.com ("CheckMyMeds"). While in theory created for patients, it is in fact an excellent tool for housestaff. It will run interactions on every drug in a patient's regimen, by brand name or generic, including many herbals; also covers food–drug interactions, rates the interactions by level of concern, describes the pharmacokinetic data for each interaction in a few lines, and finishes every cited interaction with a succinct suggestion on clinical management (e.g., lower the dose of drug A, monitor kidney function). The format allows for careful study or rapid skimming, depending on your time. It also covers significant pharmacodynamic issues, such as flagging multiple QT-prolonging drugs. While set up to help patients taking HIV meds, it works just as well on drug lists that do NOT include antiretrovirals. And it's free. Check it out.

antibiotics given for an assumed but unproven infection) after 3 days unless you document a culture-proven infection, so be aware if your hospital has such a policy.

5. *Commonly missed diagnoses*. Stumped by your patient? Consider . . .

   a. *Cardiovascular:* MI/pericarditis.

   b. *Dermatologic:* Tinea pedis/xerosis.

   c. *Endocrine:* Hypothyroidism/adrenal insufficiency.

   d. *GI:* Hepatic encephalopathy/ischemic bowel disease.

   e. *Hematologic:* DIC/ITP/TTP.

   f. *Infectious:* Meningitis/SBP/endocarditis/occult abscesses: ears, sinus, oral, pharyngeal, perirectal area/rectal fistulas/skin/soft tissue infections.

   g. *Neuro:* CNS bleeds/encephalopathy/autonomic insufficiency/neurosyphilis.

   h. *Pulmonary:* PE/DVT.

6. *Blood cultures*. Drawing blood cultures from established lines raises concern for contamination. Femoral lines are the dirtiest site.

7. *IV lines*. Of course, lines (and other invasive ports, like chest tubes) should be part of your standard daily pre-round five-point physical exam (chest, heart, abdomen, wound, and lines). Check for infiltration, thrombophlebitis, and ascending infection. Peripheral lines must be changed every 3 days. Anticipate the need for long-term indwelling lines and order them early. PICC (peripherally inserted central catheter) lines will be approved for anyone needing 14 days or more of therapy.

Line type	Life
Femoral – considered the "dirtiest" site	3–4 days maximum
Internal jugular – supposedly cleaner than fem lines, but evidence says they are equivalent	4–5 days; convention says up to 2 weeks especially if placed by interventional radiologists
Subclavian	2 weeks
PICC line	Up to 3 years!

8. *Labs*. Don't bleed patients to anemia. Make sure all the daily labs you're getting are pertinent to the patient's care, and cut down on labs and their frequency as soon as you can.
9. *Skin care*. Look for ulcers, especially in immobile patients, especially around the sacrum. Remember to check the patient's posterior daily or every other day. A good opportunity to check is when you are rounding with your team and others are present to help turn the patient over. Have a low threshold to get help from wound care or experienced nurses.
10. *Feeding*. Don't forget to feed a patient. Consider nasogastric tube (NGT)/peripheral parenteral nutrition (PPN), and, as warranted, total parenteral nutrition (TPN).
11. *Stooling*. Impaction is not a pretty thing. Patients will forget to ask for constipation treatment, so we need to ask *them*.
12. *Pain meds*. Change from IV to po ASAP. Titrating pain management with oral meds must be completed before patient can be discharged.
13. *Foley, a.k.a. urinary catheter*. If the cath has been in place for more than 5–7 days (or less, if your patient has neurologic impairment), you need to consider clamping the cath for brief periods before totally removing it. (With the Foley in place, the bladder never becomes full; neurologic signaling controlling bladder function depends on this distention to work properly.) Having to put another Foley cath in because your patient isn't able to urinate when it is removed is difficult for your patient and you. Most hospitals have their own protocols for this. Check with your nurse or the clinical nurse specialist.
14. *Self-care and feeding*. Don't forget to eat. Ask for help when you need it. Keep your sense of humor well-honed. Remember to treat others and yourself with respect and compassion. Figure out your own path to staying sane.

And never forget: Dispo, dispo, dispo. If a patient is homeless, frail, elderly, has suffered a serious event likely needing long-term convalescence, etc., give your social worker a head's up ASAP.

THE BLOOD DRAW IN 12 STEPS

Drawing blood well and safely requires practice – which is not something you get with a 2-hour tutorial a few days before being thrown into the wards. This produces students who don't feel confident in their skills and who may therefore not seek out opportunities to practice. In my mind, med students should get a half-day training in blood draws and IV placement in year 1 or 2 and have preassigned times in the ER to practice these skills. This level of instruction rarely occurs, however.

That's all the more reason you should seek out opportunities to practice procedures when you get to the wards. You should always be supervised when doing procedures, unless you're doing something you've done dozens of times. Rule of thumb: After three failed attempts, get someone else to try.

The following is a list of steps for drawing venous blood. I memorized these steps and mentally ran through them before every draw so I wouldn't forget anything.

1. *Gather materials.* Mentally run through the steps and identify the materials you'll need. They are gloves, alcohol pad, the Vacutainer® test tubes in which the blood will go, a butterfly or "direct" style needle, a yellow cup adapter for the needle, stickers with the patient's medical record number (MRN) and name, a tourniquet, a cotton ball or bandage for applying pressure to the site post-draw, an adhesive bandage, and an accessible biohazard box for disposing of the needle.

2. *Make friends with the vein* (and the patient!). This means identifying the vein you will draw.
   - Introduce yourself to the patient, explain what you will be doing, and ask for their consent and advice on a draw site. If the patient is a "frequent flyer" or IVDU, they will be able to advise you which vein has a high success rate. (Note: **The patient is always right.** In my brief clinical career, I have never seen a case where the patient was wrong, and many cases in which nurses/residents insisted on trying to draw

from veins that the patient insisted wouldn't work, much to the consternation of the patient – and to the clinician, when they failed after many attempts.) For students, the easiest and least painful sites are the basilic and cephalic veins, on the medial and lateral sides, respectively, of the antecubitum (inner elbow).

- Palpate the various options with your fingers. Note you should do this gloveless, to enhance your sensitivity. Being able to see the vein is a good sign, if it's large and slightly springy to the touch. Some little veins that are seen but not palpable are often tricky. Veins that can't be seen but can be felt, on the other hand, often work great. In other words, **feeling a vein is more helpful than seeing it.** There are several tricks to help "evoke" the veins, including rubbing and patting the potential site to warm the vessels and make them more prominent, tying on the tourniquet (temporarily!) to help engorge the veins and make them more visible, and using an adjustable lamp to light the site from the side, which will make the vessel contour more obvious. Some folks rub alcohol on the site, but since evaporation cools the skin and makes vessels shrink up, I think this hinders rather than helps.

3. *Put on gloves*. They should be comfortable – neither too tight nor loose. Double gloving can make your fingers MUCH less sensitive; I think this is overkill and reduces the chances of a safe and successful draw.

4. *Rub the site with alcohol*. My algorithm has three steps between applying alcohol and inserting the needle under the skin. There's a reason. Many phlebotomists rub alcohol on the site IMMEDIATELY before they draw blood. This is an excellent way to ensure an uncomfortable draw, since it stings like a mother. It's probably done by people who have never had their blood drawn in this fashion. LET THE ALCOHOL AIR DRY BEFORE YOU STICK. And DON'T wave your hands on it or blow on it to quicken the drying process, since it can contaminate the site. Just let it air-dry. The Golden Rule of

Procedures: "Do the procedure unto others as you would have the procedure done unto you."

5. *Label the tubes.* This is the second most important step of the draw.

6. *Assemble the needle.* I advise students to use the "butterfly" type needles, which are easier to handle and more comfortable for patients. These have a little butterfly-shaped plastic "handle" along the base of the needle, and a long thin flexible plastic tube attaching the needle to a rubber-coated "barb" that squirts out the blood. The barb needs to have a little yellow plastic cup (like a bucket with a hole in the bottom) screwed over it. Blood tubes then get plugged into the cup. The tubes get stuck into the cup with their rubber caps going in first. As the tube top touches the bottom of the cup, the barb sticks through the hole and penetrates the tube top. Since the Vacutainer tubes have a mild vacuum (thus the name), they suck blood through the butterfly needle. This is more obvious in a live demo.

7. *Apply tourniquet.* How to do this is demonstrated during your orientation training. Doing it deftly requires practice. Tip: At the beginning, I was often shy about putting the tourniquet on tightly, since I didn't want to hurt the patient. While you don't want it to hurt, and should remove and retie it if the patient asks you to, **it should be as snug as possible** – patients who I thought had no good veins were actually "easy sticks" once I started applying the tourniquet tightly, which helped me find the veins in steps 2 and 7.

8. *Uncap needle and insert.* Remember, a 45-degree angle along the course of the vein. If you don't get a "flash," don't panic. Slooooooowly pull back on the needle until it's almost (but NOT QUITE) out of the skin, and redirect the needle, again slowly, along a slightly different path. Watch for a flash at all times, and when you get it, hold the needle steady with your dominant hand and plug the tubes into the yellow cup with your other hand. Getting a flash is all about practice.

9. *Fill tubes and invert.* That is, once the tube is full, or has enough blood, pull it off the barb, invert upside down to mix

the anticoagulants, and then (ideally) place upright in a rack, or at least on its side away from any edges off which it could roll.

10. *Untie tourniquet.* If you've tied it correctly, a mild tug on the band should let it snap off.

11. *Apply cotton ball.* Or 4-by-4 or other bandage. Note: Many phlebotomists PUSH DOWN on the needle site with the cotton ball. As with the hasty alcohol application in Step 4, this is poor form: Pulling the needle out of the arm while you are pressing on the area is going to make it hurt more. Just place the cotton ball so it lightly covers the area where the needle is inserted. Once the needle is out, you can press on the cotton, and ask the patient to apply pressure to the cotton for you so you can free your hands for needle disposal.

12. *Pull out needle and place in biohazard bucket.* ***This is the most important step of the draw.*** Nothing else in the draw really matters, other than to dispose of the needle safely. Even if you don't get a flash, don't fill a single tube, whatever – it doesn't matter, as long as you avoid sticking yourself or anyone else with the needle. If you fail to draw the blood, someone else will get it. If you have a needlestick, however, it can ruin your day – or your life. (A national hotline for **needlestick post-exposure prophylaxis** is run by UCSF personnel at **1–888-HIV-4911.** Your institution may also have its own needlestick hotline.) Once the needle leaves the skin, your eyes should never completely come off of the needle until it's safely in the bucket. If other personnel are in the room with you, and the bucket is far enough away that you have to step over to it, you should announce, loudly and clearly, "I have a sharps," and keep one hand cupped along the side (**not** in front) of the needle tip. Then quickly glance to see if the path to the bucket is clear, and dispose of the needle.

13. *Apply bandage.* Thank the patient for their cooperation. Congratulations. . . . Of course, you must still fill out the lab requisition form, completely and properly. The date and time of the draw, your name, your resident's name and pager number (key, in case there's a problem), and the requested tests

should be submitted with the tubes. Ask for help if you're unsure.

PROCEDURE NOTE FORMAT

Whenever you perform a major procedure (central line, paracentesis, thoracentesis, lumbar puncture, but not routine wound dressing/packing, venous draw, or abg) you must document it in a procedure note. It should be brief. Here is an example:

1. **Procedure:** Thoracentesis
2. **Indication:** Diagnosis and treatment of pleural effusion
3. **Operator:** Ima Winner, MSIV
4. **Supervisor:** Helena Handbasket, R2, and Attending Willy Passme
5. **Preparation:** Risks, benefits, and alternatives to procedure were explained to the patient. Patient understood the rationale and gave informed consent. Sterile technique was followed using gown and gloves. Site was swathed with Beta-Dyne and a sterile field was applied. Pt was monitored on continuous pulse oximetry.
6. **Anesthesia:** 3 ml of 1% lidocaine was injected in a surface wheal and down to the pleura.
7. **Procedure:** Using a catheterized 18-G needle from the standard kit, the needle was inserted at a site 2 cm lateral to the midscapular line at the T8 level of the L back. At 2 cm depth, straw-colored fluid was obtained and noncollapsible tubing was attached to the catheter. After drawing off 10 ccs of fluid for diagnostic studies, the tubing was attached to a 1-L Vacutainer. A total of 700 cc of fluid were drawn off.
8. **Complications:** None. Pt tolerated procedure well.
9. **F/U CXR:** Stat AP CXR post-procedure showed no pneumothorax.

* * *

Dispo Dancing

Doc be nimble, Doc be quick,
D/C them patients – quite a trick!
Day and night and round-the-clock,
Let's all do the Dispo Rock![1]

So, what the heck is "dispo"? "Dispo" is short for "disposition" – that is to say, the disposition of the patient from the hospital. In a large number of cases, your patients will not be able to return to wherever they lived prior to their hospitalization. This may be because of preexisting life circumstances (e.g., patient is homeless) or the effects of the illness (e.g., frail elderly who've suffered a stroke and need prolonged physical therapy, and/or whose families can no longer take care of them, or an addicted patient who desires a shot at drug rehab).

In the beginning of wards work, students and interns may work very hard to shepherd a patient quite expeditiously through an acute illness and recovery, only to find the patient cannot be discharged owing to dispo issues. Patients may linger for as long as a week on a hospital ward despite having no true need for this level of care. This is a true bummer for all concerned: For patients, it means more time in the hospital, which puts them at risk for

[1] Sung to the tune of "Limbo Rock," by Harry Belafonte.

hospital-acquired infections, like pneumonia.[2] For students and residents, it means the team's service remains larger, with continued pre-rounding and notes and more work for the team. For the hospital, it means increased expenses.

Thus, discharging patients promptly from the hospital is a crucial skill. Unfortunately, there is utterly no formal training for students in this area and minimal training for housestaff. On the plus side, your team always has a social worker who can assist with these issues. Some wards also have a "discharge planner," whose entire job is effective dispo.

The following notes are intended to explain some basics about discharging patients. **Consider the following Appendix background reading only** – the main thing you should know is how to spot a "problem dispo patient" and get your social worker or discharge planner on the case as soon as possible. Some of the information below is taken from "Discharge Planning 101," a handout written by a discharge nurse at a UCSF facility. **Please note that discharge to hospice and discharge due to death are *not* covered below**.

Important for Discharge (D/C) Planning

- Client's acceptance of/participation in plan
- Client and family education/acceptance/participation
- Education re: all alternative D/C plans
- Client's mental status
- Client's compliance with treatment/care
- Client's drug/alcohol abuse
- Client's insurance or eligibility for insurance

---

[2] While most patients can't wait to leave the hospital, some, such as some homeless patients, get more regular meals and care on the wards than they do on the streets and may be disinclined to leave. If patients seem to have true anxiety about leaving – perhaps they're a fall risk and are afraid of being home unsupervised – this should be explored with them to identify concerns and address them. But once the obstacles have been addressed to the best of the team's ability, patients should be reminded of the health risks of staying in the hospital.

Discharge planning is a team effort beginning with the patient and involving social workers, physicians, acute care givers, family, possibly rehab therapists, dieticians, clinical nurse specialists (e.g., wound care nurse), psychiatry consult team, etc.

- Major D/C planning issues include:
  a. Home: Does patient have a permanent address?
  b. Can patient perform activities of daily living (ADLs) independently?
  c. Can patient ambulate safely? Ataxic, wide-based, or other altered gaits are unsafe.
  d. What is patient's mental status?
  e. Is patient a danger to others? Consider
    - substance abuse
    - alcohol abuse
    - psychiatric issues.
  f. What is patient's likely compliance with the rules of an accepting facility, should she or he be going someplace other than home?

A client must be "safe" for D/C. If any treatments, orders, or notes document that the patient is NOT safe, the D/C plan must be reworked.

Options. There are various types of places to which a patient may be discharged, depending on their health and circumstances. In order of intensity, they are:

1. Post-acute hospital care options: no skilled-care needs

a. **Nonstructured**
  i. *Home.* Note: Going home does not preclude having home care aides or visiting nurses. Home-bound patients with skilled-care needs (e.g., recovering from stroke) can be visited by speech, PT, or OT, as well as RNs and MSWs (social workers).

      ii. *Hotel.* Such as a single-room occupancy (SRO). No meals are provided, so client must be able to at least go out to a charity center, since cooking facilities are not on hand. Hotels are not an option for wheelchair-bound patients.

      iii. *Respite* (may stay 7 days or negotiate longer stay). Must leave after breakfast and not return until 5 P.M. Special cases – unable to walk, wheelchair bound, mental status issues – may be able to negotiate an all-day stay.

  b. **Structured.** Note: For these, clients must give all but $40/month for care from their SSI check.

      i. *Intermediate Care Facility (ICF).* Must have SSI (federal Social Security benefits for medically indigent). One LVN or RN on site for 12 hours. No home care visits allowed in most cases, since a licensed care provider is on site. Thus, not a good option if patient still needs skilled visits by ST/PT/OT/wound nurse, etc.

      ii. *Board-and-care (B&C).* Less structure than ICF, although clients of both site types may come and go as they please. No wheelchairs or walkers. B&C clients must be able to dress themselves, appear at meals by themselves, and most must be able to keep track of their own medications.

2. **Hospital-based SNF** (pronounced "sniff"; "skilled nursing facility"). For patients who still require skilled care (e.g., IV drugs) but don't require daily management on a regular ward. SNFs are for patients no longer needing daily doctor/nursing care but not ready for home. Many hospitals have SNF floors within the building – so the patient is "discharged" but still at the hospital.

a. Generally will take homeless patients if a plan for D/C for post-SNF care has been worked out prior to entry to the SNF facility (e.g., hotel, B&C).

b. Client usually must have insurance or insurance issues and are in the process of being worked out ("Medicaid pending").

c. Young clients may be difficult to place as they are often not happy with a majority of senior clients and may be less compliant than the majority of SNF residents.

d. Methadone patients may need to be negotiated with receiving institutions; rules vary.

e. Care must be such that no licensed care givers are necessary for treatment more than once a day. This means RNs as well as ST/PT/OT.

f. Visiting nurses can provide up to twice-daily outpatient care without insurance if a client is compliant and ambulatory and/or has transportation prearranged.

g. Criteria qualifying a patient as needing SNF-level care include:
   i. Needing IV antibiotics q4hr, q6hr, or q8hr
   ii. Needing dressing changes three times a day or more frequently
   iii. All rehab services
   iv. Diabetic teaching or anticoagulation – when in conjunction with other skilled needs such as wound care or PT

3. **Free-standing SNFs:** These provide subacute care, like hospital SNFs, and some have acute rehab services. They generally prefer Medicare or private insurance but occasionally accept short-term Medi-Cal patients who have a post-SNF D/C plan. All Medi-Cal and some private insurance patients require prior authorization before a free-standing SNF can be used. These SNFs often won't accept patients with compliance problems, a psych history, or methadone use. They usually won't accept a patient who may require long-term care (e.g., in persistent coma). Alternatives to a free-standing SNF include in-home support services (IHSS), adult day care, moving in with family, or 12-hour shift unskilled home care (which requires private payment).

a. *Acute rehab level of care.* This level of care is intended for patients with one or more conditions requiring intensive and

multidisciplinary care in addition to the primary condition, and
who are expected to improve with intensive therapy.

  i. Nonprimary conditions may include cognitive dysfunc-
     tion, communication disorders, incontinence, immobility,
     or dependence on others for ADLs.
 ii. To be eligible for transfer, patient's primary condition must
     be stable.
iii. Patient must be responsive to verbal or visual stimuli; i.e.,
     not be in a coma (unless the facility has a coma stimulation
     program).
 iv. Usually, the patient **must be able to tolerate three hours
     of therapy per day.**
  v. The expectation is that the patient will achieve a better level
     of function to be discharged home or to a board-and-care. If
     the patient is expected to relapse into needing a more skilled
     level of care after the rehab unit, they often will not take
     her.
b. *Subacute level of care.* This level of care is intended for patients
   with significant skilled nursing or therapist needs. This includes
   patients who:
  i. have a "trach" or tracheostomy and need continuous
     mechanical ventilation at least 50% of the day, or
 ii. have a trach and aren't on a vent but require respiratory
     therapist care, or
iii. require several of the following: total parental nutrition;
     inpatient PT/OT/ST for 2 hours a day, 5 days a week;
     tube feeding via NG tube or gastrostomy; inhalation ther-
     apy treatments four times per 24-hour period; IV therapy
     that is continuous or intermittent but frequent; debride-
     ment, wound-packing, and wound irrigation, with or with-
     out whirlpool treatment.
 iv. Examples of patients appropriate for subacute facilities
     include head trauma victims, spinal cord fracture patients
     on a vent, near-drowning survivors or others with anoxic
     brain damage, stroke survivors, those with ALS, severe

pulmonary disease – any patient who needs an intensive level of hands-on nursing care to address his or her needs.

Home therapy. Rehabilitation is often most effective and comfortable when provided in the home. Experienced therapists develop a plan and provide direct care to meet the client's rehabilitation needs. Clients and families/caregivers observe and learn skills at home where they will be used. Services include the following:

1. *Physical therapy*
   a. Restores loss of motor function and mobility.
   b. Establishes a program to maintain functional abilities.
   c. Teaches the client and family techniques for improved functional activity.
   d. Fits and trains with adaptive/assisting devices.
   e. Adapts and equips the home for safety.
2. *Occupational therapy*
   a. Restores functional capabilities in personal care and ADLs.
   b. Restores/compensates for sensory and body image lost in ADLs.
   c. Designs, fabricates, and fits adaptive/assisting devices.
   d. Teaches work simplification and energy conservation.
   e. Improves cognitive functioning.
3. *Speech therapy*
   a. Teaches alaryngeal speech.
   b. Retrains in language processing and oral speech.
   c. Augments loss by manual communication systems.
4. *Medical social work*
   a. Refers to community resources for food, medical care, housing, and financial and social needs.
   b. Counsels to minimize impediments to recovery.
   c. Explores nursing home placement when needed.

In-home supportive services. Some counties, such as San Francisco, provide funds for various services needed by chronically ill patients to allow them to remain independent in the home.

Eligibility for the services typically is determined by a social worker. Examples include:

- *Nonmedical personal services:* feeding, bed baths, dressing, bowel/bladder care, ambulation, moving in or out of bed, bathing, grooming, oral hygiene, etc.
- *Transportation to medical appointments*
- *Protective supervision:* monitor/direct activities to safeguard a mentally disoriented, impaired, or ill client from injury, hazard, or accident. Must have 24-hour need.
- *Related services:* meal preparation, meal cleanup, menu, laundry, shopping, and errands.
- *Domestic services–cleaning:* when needed in combination with the above services.

Adult day health care services. Again, San Francisco has a program for clients to attend independently operated centers providing daytime supervision for elderly or adult patients with special needs (e.g., mentally retarded). These services must have prior approval by the insurer, such as Medicaid. The patient usually must have a medical condition that requires treatment or rehab services prescribed by a physician. She must also have mental or physical impairments that affect daily living activities but that are not severe enough to require 24-hour institutional care. The expectation is that the services will maintain or improve the patient's level of function in the community, with a high potential for deterioration and institutionalization without day care.

It would be worthwhile to learn if your area offers in-home or adult day health services, which can open up discharge options for ill patients who have a home but need some support to remain in it.

* * *

APPENDIX 3

Patient Data Collection Card Templates

Included are templates for patient data collection cards. They are based on a system of cards that was popular among UCSF medical students. They should be pretty self-explanatory. The first card, originally tan, is to record basic patient data, history, and physical exam findings on admission. There is an ROS checklist as well. The second card, originally yellow, is to record labs and studies. The third card, originally blue, is for pre-rounding and daily care planning. They are the same size as standard large-size index cards.

Consider the cards as "training wheels" to get you used to data collection. Once you're in the habit, you'll have a mental image of the templates and may no longer need the actual cards.

These templates can be submitted to a copy center for photocopying onto card stock. You may have to create the mock-ups yourself. A mock-up should have the fronts and backs of the templates lined up exactly as they should align on the card stock before it gets cut into separate cards. To save paper, **two copies of the template can be placed on a page**, going horizontally rather than vertically. Make them any color(s) that works for you.

First Card Front: Basic patient data, history and physical exam findings

◎ Name:	Room:
	SSN:
MRN:	DOB:

DOA:	Contacts & Phone #'s:
DOd/c:	
☐ dictated:	CODE STATUS:_____
	SURROGATE: _____
ID/CC:	Primary: _____
	Attending: _____

HPI:

PMH:	All:
	Meds (herbals, OTCs):
PSH:	

SHx (work, housing, family, travel, ?vet): ◎

HRB: **FamHx:**
tob: drugs:
EtOH: sex:

PHYSICAL:
Gen:

Vitals: Wt: _____
T   BP   HR   RR   SaO2

HEENT:

Neck (rigidity, thyroid, JVP):

LN:

Back (CVAT):

Chest:

Card:

Abd:

Rectal:
GU:

Extr (pulses, DTRs):

Neuro (MSE CNE Mtr Sns Gait Coord)

Skin:

ROS (Y=circle; N=slash):

GEN: fever, chills, wt Δ, nt sweats, fatigue

HEENT: vision Δ, eye d/c, hearing Δ, sinus probs, epistaxis, teeth/gum probs, oral sores, sore throat, changes in voice, glasses/ contacts/ dentures

PULM: cough, sputum, hemoptysis, SOB, pleuritic CP, wheezing, recurrent bronchitis/PNA, occup. exposure (asbestos), TB, last CXR, ?DVT/PE

CARD: CP or pressure, palpitations, diaphoresis, hx: Rheum F, murmur?, syncope
  Cards risks: M$\geq$45, W$\geq$55, hx CAD, DM, PVD; fam hx early MIs; smoker; HTN; HDL<40; TChol >160; sedentary
  CHF: orthopnea, PND, pedal edema

GI: nausea, vomiting, appetite loss or Δ, diarrhea, constip, hematemesis, melena, BRBPR, Δ in BMs, PUD, GER, abd pain, dysphageia, hemorrhoids, hepatitis

GU: dysuria, hematuria, hx stones, nocturia/polyuria, incontin., UTI/pyelo
  W: menses-regularity, probs; LMP; last Pap, vag d/c, STDs, pregnancies, breast probs, last mammo
  M: hernia, testes prob, STDs, PSA

NEURO: gen. weakness, HA, sz, tremor; "dizzy"=vertigo? Pre-syncope?

MSK: joint prob, myalgias, LBP

VASC: claudication, Raynauds

ENDO: thyr. enlarged/tender, see other

HEME: anemia, bruising, clots, trnfusn

DERM: rashes, Δ in moles, itching

PSYCH: depression, anx/panic, memory Δ, hearing/seeing things

---

Templates are downloadable in color from the Cambridge University Press website at www.cambridge.org/0521676754.

Second Card Front: Record labs and studies

◎ Admit:									
Date									
Time									
WBC									
Hbg									
HCT									
Plt									
Diff									
MCV									
Retic									
Na									
K									
Cl									
Co2									
BUN									
Cr									
Glc									
Gap?									
AST									
ALT									
T bil									
D bil									
AlkP									
Alb									
Tot Prot									
Ca									
Mg									
Phos									
Lipase									
Amylase									
PT									
INR									
aPTT									
TSH									
FT4									

Second Card Back

ECG: date, findings ◎

UA: date   pH   sg   nit est prot ket glu bld WBC RBC bac cast

CXR/CT/MRI: date, findings

MICRO: date, Gram or cx, fluid type, site, growth D1   D2   D3   D4   D5

Other tests: date, findings

Date									
Time									
PH									
PaCO2									
PaO2									
Bicarb									
BE									

Third Card Front and Back: Pre-rounding and daily care planning

◎	Daily Note on:			Diet
Date	HD/POD#		Abx#	IVF/rate

Events:

Subj:

Obj-VS: Tm   Tc   BP_____   HR   RR   SaO2

(po/ng/gt + IV + misc=) I /O (=uop + BM + emesis/ngt + misc)

24 hr fluid bal: since admit: wt:

Obj-PE:

Chest-

Card-

Abd-

IV line/wound-

Obj-labs:see labsheet

A/P: <u>Problem</u>   <u>Dx A/P</u>   <u>Rx A/P</u>   Scut*

DISPO:

CODE:

THINK: △ IV line? Skin,GI ulcers? △ pain, other meds to p.o.?
   *order:=call consults, sched. studies, orders, procedures, other

* * *

APPENDIX 4

Daily Progress Note Template

Included is a template for a daily progress note. As an intern, I've noticed that while using the blue card for collecting pre-round data was fine when I carried 1–3 patients, it's less time efficient for more patients, and I've resorted to pre-rounding directly onto a full-size note. Once I finish the note, I add the daily labs to my yellow card, photocopy the note (many wards have faxes that double as copiers), pop the original in the chart, and keep the copy folded vertically in my pocket for reference. I still find the tan and yellow cards handy.

The upper right corner of the note allows you to stamp the page with the patient's ID card.

The bottom of the front and back has your name, ID code, and pager number. You can customize this template with your appropriate info, then photocopy a bunch of two-sided copies to keep on hand for pre-rounding. It saves time.

Important: The following template may need to be printed onto hospital progress notes stationery[1] – it may violate medical records rules otherwise, and your notes will be culled out of the chart. Once you've printed this onto a progress notes form (you may need to play with the formatting a bit), use that as an original and make two-sided copies for your notes.

---

[1] See Cambridge University Press website at www.cambridge.org/0521676754 for a downloadable version.

MS₄ Progress Note   **HD/POD:**   Patient
Date: **Antiobics:**   DOB
Time: **Diet:**   MRN
                             IV:

Events overnight:

Subjective:

Objective:
—**Vital Signs:**   Tm=   Tc=   BP=   HR=   RR=   SaO2=

—**In's/Out's**   po + ng/gt + IV+   / uop + stool + emesis/NGT + CT +   .

            24-hr fluid balance: wt: —**Medications**

—**Physical Exam:**   —**Labs**

    Chest:

    Card:

    Abd:

    Extr:

    Wound:

    IV lines, tubes, drains: —**Micro:** date   type   finding   .
—**Studies:**

Assessment/Plan:
_____
_____
_____

                                             MS4=Ima WINNER
                        (over)   ID#=12345678
                                             Pager#=555-1212

MS4 Progress Note, cont.	Assessment/Plan, cont.:
Date:	
Time:	

MS4=Ima WINNER
ID#=12345678
Pager#=555-1212

By the way: I've used a similar preformatted note as an intern and gotten multiple positive remarks, especially from consult services and nightfloats. The reason: They're legible. Many notes aren't. The whole point of notes is to communicate with your colleagues in case something happens while you're away. If they can't read your note, it doesn't help them. If using a preformatted note saves you time and makes your notes easy to read, use it.

* * *

APPENDIX 5

The (Don't) Panic Pages: For the Sub-I

How it's different. The role of the sub-intern/intern is very different from that of the medical student. Whereas the prized quality in a student is **thoroughness**, the prized quality in a sub-intern or intern is **EFFICIENCY**. Anything that helps you get your work done faster should be adopted, and if (like me) you're on the plodding side, you should jettison your attachment to details a bit. Conquer your work as efficiently as possible – that is the goal.

As an example, you'll see in Appendix 4 that I don't recommend pre-rounding onto cards for sub-interns, since you'll only have to recopy onto a note. Pre-round directly onto a note. If you want to keep a record, you can photocopy the note before popping it in the chart.

As a sub-I, you will have an order of magnitude more responsibility for your patients. Your resident should be working very closely with you, and expects to do so, so don't be nervous. They want to help you.

The following are some special topics I feel could bear going over, having observed UCSF sub-I's on the wards.

Sign out. Please read this section, since I have witnessed **UCSF sub-Is make multiple faux pas in giving sign out on their patients, which can easily be avoided** with a little guidance. Unlike a clerk, a sub-I signs out the overnight care of their patient to the on-call team, who (on medicine, anyway) later sign out this task to the nightfloat intern.

About 90–99 % of your sign-out consists of writing the **sign-out card**. The format is important, but so are the tasks you request your peers to perform while you are home, and how you prepare them for possible problems that may pop up on your patients. **There is an etiquette to sign out that you should know and follow**.

The card. During my residency at UCSF, we used index cards, and an example is included. These days we use a secure electronic sign-out page on a ubiquitous server. The principles of sign out, however (the what and the how), do not change whether you use a card, a digital memo, or some other method. A typical "card" looks like this:

```
                    MS4=Smith 4321
  ○                 R2=Ho 1212

JONES, Bob        12345678        Ward 5C

54 yr old Latvian-only speaking man admitted
for EtOH W/D—now off Ativan, but now in new
a fib, unsuccessful cardioversion 3/12, on
heparin gtt/Coumadin. Rate controlled w/po dilt.

PMH:          all: NKDA    meds:
Migraines                  diltiazem
EtoH-hx of sz              heparin
                           warfarin
                           TyCo#3 prn

To do:  3/13
   □6pm, MN: Adjust heparin per PTT
             (sliding scale written on back)
   □8pm: Check K, if K<3.5 give 40meq po

Probs:
   ●    Requests MSO4 for back pain.
        Written for TyCo#3; no IV pain meds!

   ●    If rapid a fib, responds to 20mg IV dilt.

   Full          IV-          Cx+
```

Notes:

--See the hole punched neatly in the upper left of the card? If you use paper, **PUNCH YOUR CARDS**! It's a pet peeve of mine, but getting sign out with cards that didn't have holes punched in them was annoying—because how the heck am I going to get your card on my ring?

--Legibility is key, so if you have to write slowly to be readable, do so. The to-do/problems section can be "revised" by placing a small white sticker over the area and writing new instructions, which is better than scratching stuff out. Rewrite your card every 3 days if you must.

--Your name and pager (first three numbers are assumed), and your R2's data. Again, legible.

--Patient's last **AND FIRST** names, and their **LOCATION**—this is key esp. when pts get moved around. It's annoying to have to track down a patient.

--HPI should be 3-4 lines. Key developments. Your resident can help you w/this. Note that pt's language ability is included along with age and sex.

--PMH should be focused on items that could come up overnight; if in doubt, include it. Some people call this section "Issues." You should note key points, e.g., see here that the PMH notes Jones has a history of seizures—key data if the pt seizes overnight. As with HPI, getting a feel for the "key" points takes experience. If in doubt, ask your R2. Allergies and key meds should also be noted.

--To do's: Should probably include the date, esp. w/a messy card. Should have a box to flag that there is a task to be done. Should include a TIME at which the task should occur. If you are asking peers to check labs at 8pm, make sure you wrote an order for those labs to be sent at 6pm. To do's should include an "if-then" statement. Don't just say "check lytes." If they're checking the K, tell them what you want them to do with the information, and under what conditions (see left).

--Probs: Anything likely to come up overnight—behavior problems, or idiosyncratic reactions to drugs, or what to do if a previous symptom/problem returns.

--Last line = code status, need for an IV, and need for cultures if spikes a fever.

   Code: if at all complicated, put note on back w/details. If pt is near death, include on back the phone #s of next of kin and possibly primary MD. If death is anticipated, you should have the "death packet" already filled out and say in the sign out where you left it—usually in your R2's mailbox, NOT the chart.

   IV: + means has to have IV access, – means if IV falls out, no need to replace.

   Cx: + means if pt spikes a fever, do the normal workup: send CXR, blood cultures times two, and UA. – means workup has been done in the last 48 hours, and there is no need to send more cultures at this time.

Again, there is an etiquette to sign out. For to-do items and problems, there are dos and don'ts:

Don't sign out anything routine that you can take care of yourself. Be aware that you are signing out to a cross-cover team that is also busy doing admissions – under all circumstances you should avoid assigning any tasks before 8 P.M. if at all possible. At 8 P.M. on UCSF medicine services, a nightfloat takes over; this is why the routine task of checking lytes for Mr. Jones, above, was assigned for 8 P.M. It means the float should take care of this.

Don't sign out complicated tasks or procedures to the cross-cover team, for similar reasons. For example, don't expect a cross-cover to fill out a PDP and discharge paperwork for a patient waiting for his or her ride home. All of that should be done well before you leave. This includes writing transfer orders for patients who are anticipated to be transferred to a new floor later that night. Also, don't sign out procedures; these may need to be done emergently/urgently but should be handled during the day by the primary team if at all possible.

Examples of common sign outs:

- "8 P.M.: Check HCT. If <30, give 2 U PRBCs."
  Common for patients with falling HCT. Note that if you sign this out, make sure a signed consent form for getting blood products is already in the chart. Also, if the patient has cardiac or fluid overload issues, it may be wise to ask the float to give the PRBCs slowly (1 unit per 4 hours) with a "Lasix chaser" (ask your R2).
- "8 P.M.: Check lytes. If K<3.5, replete by po/IV to keep at 4.0."
  See the Jones example (above). Note in this example that no amount or route is specified, but this might be done if there were issues, e.g., the patient can't tolerate po potassium and can only get IV, or vice versa (IV K is painful, so you should use po unless the level is very low, in which case use both routes simultaneously).
- "10 P.M.: Check KUB for feeding-tube placement. If in duodenum or downward in stomach, start tube feeds; feed orders

already written. If FT coiled/pointing up, give Reglan 10 mg times one and recheck KUB." Note this sign out specifies what to do under both outcomes: FT in place or not in place.

- "Midnight: Check I/O's for last 24 hrs. If not net negative 1.5 L, give 40 mg IV Lasix times one." If you check I/O's, specify a time and duration ("last 24 hrs").

Don't fail to submit a sign-out card for a patient going home. Sometimes, they stay. (More than once I had a patient fail to go home and had no sign out on them.) Sometimes, they bounce back the same night. The etiquette is to write "D/C home" or "D/C to SNF" on the card. If something goes awry, and the patient doesn't go home, the float or cross-cover will have some basic information.

For anticipated problems, you should review your sign out with your R2. I actually witnessed an MS4 sign out: "If chest pain, call cardiology fellow." This elicited some hearty chuckles from the interns. Ah, if it were only that simple! There is a "chest pain protocol" – usually to get an ECG, send a troponin, and give a nitrate (sublingual or nitropaste to chest wall). That protocol would be the standard sign out for a patient with cardiac-related chest pain. There are a range of such protocols and conventions, with variations for the specific case and situation. For the sub-I, just make sure you review the anticipated problems with your R2 before you sign out.

Don't panic – coping with emergencies. Perhaps the scenario most dreaded by MS4s is having their patient suddenly decompensate or even code. Broadly, there are two concerns: (1) Recognizing when a patient is getting into trouble, and (2) knowing what to do if things get worse – especially if it happens suddenly.

First of all, keep in mind that you are never alone in the hospital, and **YOUR MAIN JOB AS A STUDENT WITH A PATIENT "GOING SOUTH" IS TO GET YOUR SENIORS TO THE BEDSIDE PROMPTLY.**

In terms of recognition, let's start with total catastrophe: a code blue. This is often easiest, since in a full code the code team will be taking care of business and you are there simply to help. In such situations, you should start off by following your basic life support (BLS) training.

The role of the medical student in a code blue. When would this come up? If your patient suddenly should lose consciousness IN FRONT OF YOU, *immediately* approach them, shake them, and ask loudly: "Mr. Jones, are you okay?" Feel for a radial pulse and check for breathing. If they (1) are not waking up despite aggressive shaking, (2) are not breathing, or (3) their pulse is absent, *and they have a full or partial code status*, then they are a code blue.[1] Shout out the door, "CODE BLUE! CODE BLUE! CALL A CODE!" This will bring the nurses running as well as the code team. NEVER LEAVE THE BEDSIDE, at least not until the physician running the code is present, takes over, and gives you some other task to do.

As the nurses and other staff arrive, your immediate job in the next 60 seconds is to assist the staff in assessing and stabilizing the ABCs – airway, breathing, circulation. **Check for bilateral breath sounds, and feel for a femoral pulse**. Staff should be getting vitals, including a *manual* blood pressure, and should be slapping defibrillator pads on the patient. There will inevitably be non-code personnel hanging around outside the door. Point to one of them and say: "You! Please get me this patient's chart!" Use their name if you know it. (In a code, it is imperative to direct commands to specific people; resist the temptation to shout, "Somebody get me the chart.")

As soon as the code team arrives, your job, as the primary person following the patient, will be to give a succinct bullet about the patient to the resident running the code: their age, major medical

---

[1] On the other hand, if you *come upon* them unconscious, they could just be sleeping, or very sedated. If they're breathing and have a good pulse, you're almost certainly not looking at a code situation – but you should still be able to arouse them. If you can, but their vitals are poor, it's a pseudo-code. If you can't, but vitals are stable, you're looking at an urgent change in status – don't call a code, but contact your senior immediately.

problems, and the events immediately preceding their decompensation. Hopefully, someone will have brought you the chart to help you check specific information if the code team has questions.

Once seniors from your team arrive, they often take over as the primary informants, but you should listen closely to assist with this responsibility. You may be given some other assignment by the code resident. If you are no longer needed for information, and no one is giving you a job, take it upon yourself to help – you can offer to relieve the person administering chest compressions, for example, or take it upon yourself to obtain an arterial blood gas. Again, DO NOT LEAVE THE BEDSIDE unless one of your seniors gives you a task. You may be needed to answer a question.

Somewhat trickier – the pseudo-code. The term *pseudo-code* applies to situations in which a patient is not (yet) a code – i.e., not in shock (low blood pressure with altered mental status or organ injury), cardiac arrest (pulseless), or respiratory failure (not breathing or oxygenating) – but is looking rapidly worse. Altered vitals with loss of consciousness is a code; altered vitals but still conscious is a pseudo-code. For example, a patient whose shortness of breath is getting worse and appears distressed with more labored breathing or a patient who is complaining of feeling unwell with a falling blood pressure. They are still talking, but look bad, and their vitals are so-so: a systolic blood pressure in the 90s, a heart rate over 100, respiratory rate in the mid-30s, or oxygen sats below 92 % despite escalating use of oxygen and masks.

First: Remain calm. If things get really bad, you can always call a code. Meanwhile, your goal is to try to avert that outcome, if possible.

Second: Your main job is to get your senior to the bedside as quickly as possible. While you are waiting, get a few tasks underway. In the pseudo-code, as in a code, do not leave the patient's bedside if they look sick enough to worry you. Ask personnel to come into the room to help you, and (politely) **assign someone else the task of paging your senior** with the urgent message, "Mr. Jones is sick; need help, please come immediately."

In a pseudo-code, prompt action may avoid a full-blown code blue. Often the pseudo-code ends with the patient being transferred to a higher level of care (e.g., ICU). If vital signs become deranged enough that the patient loses consciousness or becomes unresponsive, or your team needs additional help to stabilize the patient, a formal code blue may be called.

While you are waiting for your senior, it is often appropriate to use what I call "**The Cheech[2] of Badness**": Get a set of vitals, order a stat portable chest x-ray and ECG, and obtain stat abg, CBC, and lytes. In virtually all significant decompensations, all of these tests would be obtained anyway, whether you wind up diagnosing an MI, PE, abdominal catastrophe, status asthmaticus, etc. Except in a COPD patient with known CO_2 retention and hypoxic drive (a "retainer"), in which case you should aim for a sat of about 93%, it is never wrong to give oxygen.

A pseudo-code often looks exactly like a code blue, but at a slower pace. Unlike in a code, the patient is often still conscious, and probably very anxious – so give your orders briskly, but calmly. When your senior arrives, describe your concerns, the latest vitals, what tests you ordered (or results, if you're starting to get them), and your assessment. Your senior will take over from there.

Psychological Survival. The sub-I is like a mini-internship, and can be quite intense. Fortunately, it's short, and there's time later in the fourth year to recover (unlike internship!). As someone who garnered a reputation as "The Happy Intern" during my MR1 year, I have some tips for psychological survival.

1. **It's tough. Admit it**. One way to survive is to acknowledge the stresses you're feeling. Being a sub-I or an intern is a high-stress job. Every day as an intern, I woke up and told myself, "It's an impossible job; I'm doing the best I can." It may be

---

[2] *cheech* (chēech), n. UCSF medicine slang for any conventional diagnostic algorithm. For example, the "fever cheech" involves obtaining a chest film, urinalysis, and two peripheral blood cultures.

macho to pretend it's no biggie, but the truth is that this job is a bitch. In my third month of internship I seemed to find myself crying in the bathtub every other night, telling my partner I wasn't going to survive and wondering how the hell I could quit now. (And this from "The Happy Intern"!) So, admit that it's hard. Going home and crying about your experiences on the wards doesn't make you a wuss – it's normal and typical. Verbalizing your stresses and having a friend or family member to whom you vent your frustrations can be very healing. It's when we *can't* talk about problems that they have the greatest power over us. As we used to say in ACT UP, "Silence equals death."

2. **Have a restorative practice**. I was going to write, "Have a spiritual practice," but I realized that some folks may have practices that restore them without considering them "spiritual."[3] This means things like meditation or prayer, but also things like getting a massage, watching *Buffy the Vampire Slayer* every week, or cooking kim-chee for your family. Anything that you find enjoyable and will help you take your focus off the wards for a few hours qualifies.

3. **Have an exercise regimen**. For some this also qualifies as their "restorative practice," but for those who don't get regular exercise, I swear to you: Physical stress relief is as important as mental stress relief. It will help your sleep cycle, your digestion, your moods – in ways that endless amounts of *Buffy* and kim-chee can't. Just do it.

4. **Have a ritual for coping with death**. If you haven't had a patient die as an MS3, you will almost certainly have that experience as an MS4. Many students find themselves struggling

---

[3] And for those who get twitchy at any mention of terms like "spirituality" in the scientific enterprise of medicine: Don't wig. Even utter atheists can agree that the business of helping patients heal often puts us in touch with the potential magnificence of human beings. So, if you want to mentally substitute "awareness" or "humanism" or "beneficence" where other folks may use "spirituality," go for it. There's no point in quibbling over terms – committed practitioners of medicine, regardless of our vocabulary choices, are on the same team.

with guilt, sadness, and even anger after a patient's death. Some are shocked at how their seniors barely acknowledge the event and seem to have totally forgotten it by the end of the day. Yes, that does happen, and yes, it is weird, but often it's necessary if you're not going to get taken under by the weight of the work. The truth is, the rest of our patients, and their needs, don't go away, no matter what else is going on. We need to keep working. On the other hand, we also need to mark what has occurred.

At UCSF, some housestaff get together once a year for a dinner to remember their patients who've died. Other people say a prayer or fold a crane. When I have a patient who's dying, I call my partner at home and ask him to make a light offering to Buddha. Whatever helps you cope, or makes the experience meaningful – do it. You'll feel better.

* * *

Eliciting the Code Status: A Very Important Job That We Doctors Do Very Badly

The problem. Talking with patients about end-of-life care, advance directives, and code status – a.k.a. "the code talk" – is a task shared by most inpatient physicians. Despite the frequency with which we face this task, most physicians don't feel comfortable or competent doing it. **Talking about the code status often is done badly, if done at all.** Thus, it may be no surprise that two-thirds of patients admitted to the hospital do not have a conversation with medical staff about their code status[1] – despite the fact that most patients *want* to have this conversation. In this discussion, the term "code talk" refers to the initial conversation at the time of admission, but in truth, the "talk" may be a series of discussions with staff over the hospital stay.

Why do we even bother to have a code talk with patients? **Because sometimes a full-bore resuscitation does not make sense,** either because the patient does not wish to be put through the pain and trauma of a resuscitation, or because his chances of surviving a code are vanishingly small. In those cases, the code status may be "do not resuscitate" (DNR) or some form of a "limited code," such as "no shocks or chest compressions, pressors okay." Often, residents have an interest in avoiding a code blue in a patient who does not want it or is not expected to survive it.

---

[1] Frank C, Heyland DK, Chen B, et al. Determining resuscitation preferences of elderly inpatients: a review of the literature. *CMAJ*. 2003;169:795–799.

Effective communication with patients about advance directives is challenging under the best circumstances – i.e., when you are the primary provider, know the patient well, talk about it when the patient is in good health, and have plenty of time to answer questions. In most cases, residents discuss code status with patients they've just met, who are significantly or critically ill, with very little time.

Why we avoid the talk. As an admitting medical student or resident, reasons you might avoid the code talk with your patient include ignorance, inexperience, or the belief that it will upset the patient or is not worth the time.

Few students will have seen even *one* code blue. Thus, you may not know the practical issues around resuscitation preferences, such as what interventions or technologies are involved, the decision points the team likely will face during the code, or – what patients really want to know – their chances of surviving. You can hardly explain these issues if you're unfamiliar with them yourself. The basics are covered herein, to help get you started.

Just as important as technical ignorance: You likely will have had few, if any, chances of observing your seniors talk with patients about their code status – much less, see them do it well. Your seniors may be no more comfortable bringing up this subject than you are. Physician discomfort and lack of time are two major reasons why doctors avoid discussing code status with patients.[2]

Some providers believe patients find the subject of code status upsetting: "Why are you asking me about this? Do you think I'm going to die here in the hospital, Doctor?" It should be made clear to patients that you have this conversation with every admitted patient and that you simply want to document their wishes for the medical record. In a review of forty-five studies on the subject, it was found that most patients (45–100%) were comfortable having

---

[2] Layton R, Adelman H, Wallach P, et al. Discussions about the use of life-sustaining treatments: a literature review of physicians' and patients' attitudes and practices. *J Clin Ethics*. 1994;5:195–203.

discussions about CPR.[3] Moreover, physicians often are mistaken in their guesses about patients' CPR preferences – in the SUPPORT study, mistaken 50% of the time.[4]

Eliciting at least a preliminary code status can be done reasonably quickly and at least as competently as eliciting informed consent for a procedure – something most doctors agree is a legal and ethical responsibility. The code talk should be seen in a similar light. In one study,[5] the code talk took a mean of 10 minutes – less time than it takes to insert a central line. If the talk winds up avoiding a code in a person with little chance of success and/or gives her more control, more peace, and less pain at the time of death, it is worth it.

Vocabulary. The subject of resuscitation is awash with jargon and often confusing for housestaff, not to mention the patients.

Advance directive: A legal document in which the patient states what kind of care he would like to have *if he becomes unable to make medical decisions* (e.g., it kicks in if the patient becomes comatose or delirious). In the U.S., laws governing advanced directives vary by state. Patients may cite types of treatment they do not wish to have, or that they insist on having, in case they cannot communicate that desire at the time of care. Advanced directive documents can be used in conjunction with a surrogate decision maker designated in a durable power of attorney document (DPOA).

Code blue: Synonym for a resuscitation. A code blue is called when a patient becomes unresponsive, usually because they have lost a pulse, become hypotensive (shock), or stopped breathing. Resuscitation is performed to revive or stabilize patients who otherwise are expected to die, imminently. Every hospital has a

---

[3] Frank C, Heyland DK, Chen B, et al. Determining resuscitation preferences of elderly inpatients: a review of the literature. *CMAJ.* 2003;169:795–799.

[4] Teno JM, Hakim RB, Knaus WA, et al. Preferences for cardiopulmonary resuscitation: physician-patient agreement and hospital resource use. *J Gen Intern Med.* 1995;10:179–186.

[5] Tulsky JA, Chesney MA, Lo B. How do medical residents discuss resuscitation with patients? *J Gen Intern Med.* 1995;10:436–442.

"code team" composed of staff from medicine, anesthesia, surgery, pharmacy, and nursing; these staff rush to the location of the patient when the code blue is called. The protocol for resuscitation is laid out in the American Heart Association's *Advanced Cardiac Life Support* (ACLS) manual, and may include interventions such as

- *Rapid-sequence intubation:* insertion of an endotracheal tube (ET tube) or other device to stabilize an airway in a patient too mentally impaired to protect his airway himself or whose airway may be lost due to swelling from an allergic reaction, etc.
- *Assisted ventilation:* use of a bag-valve mask or ventilator machine to help a patient breathe when she is not taking breaths on her own, or is hypoxic despite her own respiratory effort.
- *Defibrillation:* use of electric shocks to try to bring a patient out of ventricular fibrillation or pulseless ventricular tachycardia, two kinds of fatal heart rhythms. Lower joules of electrical energy may be used to shock a patient out of rhythms such as ventricular tachycardia or atrial fibrillation with rapid ventricular response; this is called *cardioversion*. The electrical energy is delivered via pads stuck to the sternum and back/lateral chest wall or by paddles held onto the chest manually.
- *Chest compressions:* pushing on a patient's chest wall to circulate her blood if she lacks a strong pulse of her own (usually determined by palpating the femoral pulse in the groin).
- *Pressor medications:* typically, arginine vasopressin, epinephrine, neosynephrine, dopamine, etc., to maintain blood pressure in patients with shock (i.e., low blood pressure resulting in loss of consciousness or end-organ damage).

To "call a code" can mean initiating a code blue resuscitation; it can also mean to declare an end to resuscitation efforts (e.g., "It's been 25 minutes; do you want to call the code?").

Code status: The patient's prior stated preference for resuscitation measures. For "full code" patients, all possible interventions will be used until the patient is stabilized or dies. For DNR patients, no resuscitation efforts will be employed and no code should be called if they have a sudden loss of responsiveness. For patients with in-between statuses a code is called, but some interventions may be specifically barred.

Competence: A legal concept. When courts declare an adult "incompetent," it means the person does not have the capacity to make informed decisions, usually about *all* aspects of life, including medical decisions. In modern medical practice, physicians often make de facto determinations that a patient lacks decision-making capacity for medical matters without consulting a court. The modern consensus is that a person has medical decision-making capacity if they can give informed consent, i.e., they can explain their diagnosis and prognosis; the nature of the treatment options; the risks, benefits, and alternatives to each option; and likely consequences of their choice.[6] See *Decision-making capacity*.

CPR: Cardiopulmonary resuscitation. Measures taken to stabilize a patient with cardiac or respiratory failure. See *Code blue*.

Decision-making capacity: When a patient refuses a treatment that is strongly recommended (e.g., cardiac angiogram for an ST-elevation myocardial infarction), and especially if he has a condition that may affect decision-making ability such as dementia, schizophrenia, or depression, an assessment of decision-making capacity is in order. Patients have decision-making capacity if (1) they can make and communicate a choice; (2) they can give informed consent (see *Competence*); (3) their decisions are consistent with their values and goals; (4) their decisions do not stem from a delusion; and (5) they use reasoning to make their choice.[7]

DNI: "Do not intubate." A code status that lies somewhere between full code and total DNR. While technically a patient may opt for "DNI/resuscitation okay," in reality this status may be tricky to accommodate. See below.

---

[6] Lo B. Decision-making capacity. In: *Resolving Ethical Dilemmas: A Guide for Clinicians*. Philadelphia: Lippincott Williams & Wilkins; 2000:80–88.

[7] Ibid.

DNR: "Do not resuscitate." A code status in which resuscitation measures are not undertaken should the patient have an abrupt life-threatening event. Please note that "DNR" is not equivalent to "comfort care" (see *Goals of care*). Many prefer to use the terms *Do Not Attempt Resuscitation* and DNAR, since this makes explicit to patients that undergoing resuscitation is no guarantee of survival (see below).

DPOA: Durable power of attorney. Can refer to the surrogate decision maker or to the document that designates her. See *Durable power of attorney for health care decisions.*

Durable power of attorney for health care decisions: A durable power of attorney (DPOA) is another kind of advance directive. A DPOA states whom a patient has chosen to make health care decisions for herself. It becomes active any time the patient enters a state in which she is unable to make medical decisions. A DPOA is generally more useful than other forms of advance directives.

Futility: Applies to medical interventions that would serve no meaningful purpose. Physicians may justify withholding treatments due to futility if (1) the requested treatment has no pathophysiologic rationale, such as a patient requesting an antibiotic that has no activity against his particular infection; (2) the patient is experiencing progressive shock in the face of maximal treatment, in which case CPR would not be effective; or (3) the treatment has already failed in the patient. Beyond these scenarios, declaring efforts to be "futile" is often problematic. In the literature, futility applies to interventions with less than a 1% chance of success – which in practice covers very few cases.[8]

Goals of care: Specifically, whether a patient wishes to pursue treatment focused mainly on cure or control of disease, treatment focused on pain and symptom control (a.k.a. "palliative care," "comfort care," or "hospice care"), or something in between. Usually, a comfort care strategy involves a DNR designation. On the other hand, a DNR status does not necessarily mean comfort care; terminally ill patients may wish aggressive treatment of disease

[8] Lo B. Futile interventions. In: *Resolving Ethical Dilemmas: A Guide for Clinicians.* Philadelphia: Lippincott Williams & Wilkins;2000:72–79.

while also wishing to avoid a code should they have a sudden life-threatening event.

Guardian: A court-appointed surrogate for patients who do not have a designated surrogate, who have multiple first-degree relatives who cannot agree on a treatment plan, or who have a surrogate clearly acting in his own interest instead of the patient's.

Living will: One type of advance directive. It only comes into effect when a patient is terminally ill. Being terminally ill generally means a patient's prognosis is fewer than 6 months to live. In a living will, patients describe the kind of treatment they want in certain situations, but do not designate a surrogate.

Resuscitation: See *Code blue.*

Surrogate decision maker: Any person who makes decisions for a patient who lacks decision-making capacity. If the person was specifically designated by the patient, the surrogate is termed a *proxy;* if designated in a DPOA document, the surrogate is termed the *DPOA.* A court-appointed surrogate is a *guardian* or *conservator.* The next of kin may assist the team in determining the patient's wishes, if no advance directives or DPOA exists to assist with decision making.

What is your job? You want to finish your code talk with, at minimum, two pieces of information: (1) a code status and (2) the name and phone number of the person the patient would want making decisions for her, if she gets too sick to tell us herself – in other words, a surrogate decision maker. This does not have to be a certified DPOA, but if the patient has one, so much the better. Code information can be gathered by the end of the initial history and physical exam.

For young persons with illnesses easily treated, the appropriateness of a "full code" designation is self-evident and many housestaff would not even discuss it. However, **even a patient who is expected to do well may wind up in a condition in which they lack decision-making capacity.** Thus, discussion (or, if you prefer, confirmation) of full code status, and designation of a surrogate, still applies. For patients with severe acute illness, comorbid conditions (especially cardiovascular or pulmonary disease), terminal illness, or very debilitated or elderly patients, exploration of CPR preferences makes even more sense.

In a perfect world, patients discuss CPR with their primary care provider before they come to the hospital – but this is rarely the case. Often you will be the first medical provider to have this conversation with the patient. In most cases, your talk is the beginning of an ongoing discussion the patient will have with medical personnel. Thus, you may admit a patient who has a very low chance of surviving a code, for whom the code status remains the default "full code" – at least until the patient has some time to discuss it with his family and/or primary care provider. That may not be optimal, but it is acceptable. The code status in such cases, however, should be revisited with the patient, family, and/or primary as time and the evolving course warrant.

When it gets complicated: Not full-code. If a patient designates himself full code, he is choosing a position that is the default position anyway. The appropriateness of a full-code status can be called into question based on circumstances but rarely leads to medicolegal issues for the admitting team, in the short-term.

On the other hand: Sometimes, a patient will surprise an interviewer by expressing a desire to be made DNR, when this has never been discussed with her doctors before. In such cases, **you must satisfy yourself that the patient has decision-making capacity** – i.e., can give informed consent, has a position consistent with her values (hard to know unless you're in touch with family, friends, or primary), is not having delusions, and is using reason to arrive at her decision. Keep in mind that **a patient can have decision-making capacity but still not have accurate understanding of her prognosis or resuscitation technologies** – in which case the appropriateness of her choice may be questioned (see the following discussion).

What if the patient's depressed? A new designation of DNR should be gauged against a surrogate or primary's opinion as to whether this preference is consistent with the patient's values at a time when he was *not* depressed. If this is not possible, a psychiatric consultation may be needed to determine a diagnosis of depression and the validity of the DNR order. The difference between acceptance of a terminal condition and depression can be difficult to ascertain.[9]

If a patient is DNR or some status other than full code, be aware that **most hospitals will have a special form** for the order placed at the front of the chart, usually requiring an attending's signature. You may wish to bring this form to rounds for the attending to sign right away. **If there is any question about the appropriateness of a DNR or partial code status, the status should be full code until the questions are clarified.**

"Why didn't you just shock him?" The challenge of patient ignorance. The challenges of the code talk are similar to those behind eliciting informed consent for a procedure – meaning that for the consent or code status to be valid, the patient must demonstrate an understanding of the basic concepts involved. For patients to express a preference about their code status, they need some simple explanations of what is involved in a code blue.

Thanks to television shows like *ER*, patients have some very funny ideas about resuscitation.[10] For example, most codes on TV are successful, whereas most codes in real life are not. A patient may have the mistaken idea that "bringing me back to life" is as easy as throwing a switch. Indeed, I remember a conversation with the young nephew of a patient on my service who, after several weeks, finally succumbed to late-stage AIDS, cirrhosis, and sepsis with multi-organ failure. As I was giving my condolences to the family, the child pulled on the sleeve of my white coat and asked, "Doctor, why didn't you just shock him?" After a second of stunned silence, I said, "Because, honey, his body was so tired it wouldn't have done any good – he would have just died all over again. It was time for us to let him go." That seemed to satisfy him.

[9] Heller M. End of life care and advanced directives. [Oral presentation], UCSF. April 12, 2004.

[10] Diem SJ, Lantos JD, Tulsky J. Cardiopulmonary resuscitation on television: miracles and misinformation. *N Engl J Med.* 1996;334:1578–1582.

Advance directives rarely let you off the hook. I have found few advance directive documents that are written in a manner practical for physicians. Patients often express preferences that are unsurprising – e.g., they do not wish to be maintained on ventilation "if my condition is deemed futile by my doctors." The problem with such a vague directive is that there is no standard for determining futility – should we declare failure after 2 weeks, or 2 months? (UCSF Moffitt Hospital has seen plenty of patients on vents for at least that long, if not much longer.) Some patients who declare themselves DNI may in fact have conditions, such as asthma, that can be quickly reversed within a couple of days, if not hours, on a ventilator – but they refuse intubation because they think it means they will remain on a vent forever.

The bottom line: Patients and families, even when they have advance directives, often lack basic information about CPR techniques. They need simple explanations of these concepts, as well as real facts about the risks and success rates of resuscitation, to give informed consent.

How to do it. Discussing the code status can be done during the initial history and physical. Some consider it part of the history, like the social history. Others ask about it after finishing the physical exam. Keep in mind that the code talk may be had with a family member if the patient obviously lacks decision-making capacity (i.e., not communicating, not able to reason or understand due to delirium or mental illness, etc.).

First tenet: **Avoid jargon.** Don't say "ET tube," say "breathing tube." Don't say "pressors," say "strong medicines to restart the heart and maintain your blood pressure." Don't say "code blue," say "CPR" – up to 80% of patients and families have heard of CPR.[11]

One way to avoid slipping into jargon is to imagine the patient is a close, nonmedical friend or relative. (I pretend I'm explaining

---

[11] Frank C, Heyland DK, Chen B, et al. Determining resuscitation preferences of elderly inpatients: a review of the literature. *CMAJ*. 2003;16:795–799.

something to my grandmother.) Since we don't usually use technical language with our loved ones, this mental trick can help you avoid accidentally using Doctorese with your patient.

Second tenet: **Be complete.** One study on how residents discussed code status with patients found that while all the physicians mentioned mechanical ventilation, only 55% mentioned chest compressions and 32% mentioned intensive care.[12] What you want to know from the patient are answers to the following questions:

1. Have they ever talked about CPR with their doctor? If so, do they have a signed advance directive or a durable power of attorney? (If so, find out how to get a copy.)
2. If they stop breathing on their own, how do they feel about the insertion of a breathing tube and use of a breathing machine (i.e., a ventilator)?
3. If their heart should suddenly stop, how do they feel about receiving shocks, chest compressions, and/or strong medicines to try to restart their heart?
4. Have they ever discussed their medical preferences with a friend or loved one? (If yes, get the name and contact information.)
5. If they got so sick in the hospital that they could not tell us what they wanted, whom would they want us to ask about their medical decisions? (Again, get the name and contact information.)

Third tenet: **Use statistics.** Only 13% of the physicians in the Tulsky study mentioned the patient's likelihood of survival after CPR, and no physician used a numerical estimate.

Of patients undergoing CPR <u>in the hospital</u>, 13% survive to discharge.[13] CPR is *most* effective in people who have reversible

[12] Tulsky JA, Chesney MA, Lo B. How do medical residents discuss resuscitation with patients? *J Gen Intern Med.* 1995;10:436–442.

[13] Ebell MH, Becker LA, Barry HC, et al. Survival after in-hospital cardio-pulmonary resuscitation. A meta-analysis. *J Gen Intern Med.* 1998;13:805–816.

diseases or who have a witnessed heart rhythm disturbance while hospitalized (e.g., shocking a heart attack patient out of ventricular fibrillation). CPR is *least* effective in people who suffer an unwitnessed event or an event *outside* the hospital, in the setting of chronic diseases such as sepsis, renal failure, or heart failure.[14] Patients who, at baseline, spend more than half their time in bed have a 2–3% chance of survival to discharge after CPR.[15] Cancer patients with an *unexpected* sudden cardiac event had a 22% chance of survival to discharge after CPR,[16] whereas cancer patients with *anticipated* arrests due to progressive disease unresponsive to treatment had a 0–2% chance of survival to discharge. Surprisingly, neither metastatic cancer nor age per se predicted the success of CPR.[17]

In one study of more than 800 patients who survived CPR *in the hospital* to discharge, 75% were independent in their daily life afterward, while 17% had lasting cognitive impairment.[18]

Fourth tenet: **Use active listening.** This means, if you are talking more than two-thirds of the time, probably you're not listening enough. Two basic techniques of active listening are "restating" and "reflection." In **restating**, you rephrase what a patient just told you, to show you understand the content. Restating begins with phrases such as, "So, correct me if I'm wrong, but what I hear you saying is . . ." or "In other words, you believe that . . ." In **reflection**, you are ascertaining the *emotions* around what was said, rather than content: "Sounds like you have some strong

[14] O'Keeffe S, Redahan C, Keane P, et al. Age and other determinants of survival after in-hospital cardiopulmonary resuscitation. *Quarterly J Med.* 1991;81:1005–1010.

[15] Vitelli C, Cooper K, Rohatko A, et al. Cardiopulmonary resuscitation and the patient with cancer. *J Clin Oncol.* 1991;9:111–115.

[16] Ewer MS, Kish SK, Martin CG, et al. Characteristics of cardiac arrest in cancer patients as a predictor of survival after CPR. *Cancer.* 2001;92:1905–1912.

[17] Varon J, Walsh GL, Marik PE, et al. Should a cancer patient be resuscitated following an in-hospital cardiac arrest? *Resuscitation.* 1998;36:165–168.

[18] de Vos R, de Haes HC, Koster RW, et al. Quality of survival after cardiopulmonary resuscitation. *Arch Intern Med.* 1999;159:249–254.

feelings about being intubated," which can be followed with, "Tell me more about that." Reflection can help uncover and address false understandings about CPR very effectively.

Fifth tenet: **Establish the goals of care.** In the Tulsky study, 90% of the time physicians failed to ask about the patients' values and goals of care – basic information needed to assess the validity of a code status. Patients with irreversible Class IV heart failure or end-stage cirrhotic liver disease may have a very low quality of life and a prognosis equivalent to metastatic cancer; they may be ready to discuss hospice care, which would include DNR status. In fact, your quick admission code talk may lead to an appropriate change in their declared goals of care.

The following are some vignettes related to giving the code talk. I offer these not because I necessarily see you, as a medical student, undertaking complex conversations like these on your own (at least not early on). But I want to give you a sense of what code talks look like and what sorts of questions come up. In real life, if a patient raises a question or issue you don't feel you can address, simply say, "That's a good point, and I have questions about that myself. Why don't I ask my resident to come talk to you about that further?"

What if the code status is "wrong"? I noted some situations in which the validity of a new declaration of DNR status may be questioned – e.g., if a patient is depressed and his position contradicts his previously expressed views. You should also carefully question a patient with good odds of a successful resuscitation who declares herself DNR. She may have mistaken beliefs about what it means to have CPR or to be on a ventilator. As noted, a myocardial infarction patient on telemetry who has a witnessed dysrhythmic event has a good chance of surviving a code to discharge. Such patients may be counseled to consider favoring resuscitation.

Having DNR status does not automatically bar a patient from having surgery, but it should be clarified with the patient, family, and primary whether the DNR status is suspended during the surgery and immediate post-op period, as is often the convention.

You may also encounter situations in which a patient has a very low chance of surviving a code blue, and yet the patient or her family desires a full-code status, even after counseling about the dismal odds. An attending may insist on the futility of a full code and may have the legal right to make the patient DNR anyway. By the strict definition of the medical ethics literature, futility is <1% chance of success, which may indeed be the odds of surviving a code to discharge for certain patients (see the statistics cited previously).

More problematic situations arise when patients choose a code status somewhere between "full" and "DNR," which may be allowed in some hospitals. Such "limited codes" or "limited aggressive therapy"[19] orders can be problematic for code teams, since events in a code are often unpredictable and there is not enough time to gather the facts before actions must be taken.

One example: A patient declares himself DNI ("do not intubate") but resuscitation is authorized. This is tricky, since most patients requiring resuscitation will have altered mental status if not frank coma. They cannot protect their airway and will likely aspirate and risk death if they are not intubated. Thus, this status can be argued as untenable. Some patients who request "DNI" status have been on a ventilator in the past, which may be the basis for their reluctance to be intubated again. That may be okay, so long as they understand they may not survive a code without intubation. DNI status in someone who has never been intubated should result in close questioning of the patient to make sure his refusal is based on a clear understanding of the issues and the likely repercussions of that decision.

For more reading on this subject, see Bernard Lo's chapter on DNR orders in *Resolving Ethical Dilemmas*.[20]

[19] Choudry NK, Choudry S, Singer PA. CPR for patients labeled DNR: the role of the limited aggressive therapy order. *Ann Intern Med.* 2003;128:65–68.

[20] Lo B. Do not resuscitate orders. In: *Resolving Ethical Dilemmas: A Guide for Clinicians*. Philadelphia: Lippincott Williams & Wilkins; 2000:147–155.

Code Talk Vignette 1: "We Thought She Was Getting Better." Mrs. C is a 64-year-old English-speaking Chinese American woman with a diagnosis of perihilar cholangiocarcinoma. She has a son and daughter who live near her. She had surgery 8 weeks ago and, although quite jaundiced and fatigued, was functioning independently at home. Two days ago she began having fevers. This morning her daughter came to check on her and found her in bed, diaphoretic and delirious. Upon arrival in the ER she is found to have a blood pressure of 80/40, pulse 135 bpm, platelets of 50,000/mm³, and elevated coagulation tests suggestive of severe disseminated intravascular coagulation, probably due to septic shock. After obtaining central venous access, the resident gives several liters of IV fluids, then starts first one and then a second pressor. Still, the mean arterial pressure remains at the tenuous level of 60 mm Hg. The resident approaches her daughter to discuss her status.

Comments

RESIDENT: Ms. C?

DAUGHTER: Yes?

RESIDENT: I'm Dr. X, I'm taking care of your mother.

DAUGHTER (*anxious*): How is she?

RESIDENT: She is gravely ill. Her blood pressure is very low and she appears to be in septic shock. In other words, we think she has a bacterial infection in her blood, probably related to her cancer, and that is causing the shock, or low blood pressure.

Notice that the resident realizes the daughter may not know what "septic shock" is, so explains in other terms. Using jargon is often unavoidable, but if you catch yourself doing it, try to repeat what you've said in simpler language right away.

DAUGHTER: But she's going to get better, right? You can treat it with antibiotics?

RESIDENT: We can treat her infection with antibiotics, yes, but the infection is releasing poisons into her blood that are damaging her organs. We have had to give her strong medicines to maintain her blood pressure, but it looks like she is getting worse. She is as sick as someone who has been hit by a car. It is painful for me to tell you this, but there is a strong chance your mother will not survive this.

DAUGHTER: I don't understand – we thought she was getting better. The surgeon said she did very well with the surgery. She could die?

RESIDENT (*nodding*): Yes, she could very well die. Sounds like this comes as a shock. As you know, your mother has a very bad cancer – only about 10% of patients survive five years after surgery. They can get blood infections, just like your mother has. Did your mother ever discuss her preferences about CPR with you or her doctors?

DAUGHTER (*puzzled*): CPR?

RESIDENT: Yes, "cardiopulmonary resuscitation" – meaning things like whether she'd want a breathing tube to help her breathe, or shocks or chest compressions to help revive her if her heart stopped working. Sometimes people write out their preferences in a document called an "advance directive" or a "living will."

DAUGHTER (*looking dazed*): Uh, not that I know of. I mean, no, I don't think she has a living will. No one brought it up.

RESIDENT: So, she never officially designated a "durable power of attorney" to make decisions for her, if she got sick? And she never talked to you or other family about what she'd want if something like this happened?

Comparing the condition of a septic shock patient to a car accident victim may seem strange, but it is a way for laypersons to quickly get a concrete sense of the risk of death their loved one may face.

"Sounds like this comes as a shock" – use of reflection.

Where did the resident get this survival statistic? Before talking to the family, he quickly checked UptoDate for prognosis of patients with her cancer type – it took four minutes, but greatly affects how the daughter sees her mother's situation.

Task 1: Ask about prior discussion with doctors re: CPR preference.

It is surprisingly common for the doctors of patients with cancer to avoid discussing code status – despite the fact that such patients have a significant chance of facing the sort of situations in which advance directives and DPOAs are most helpful.

Tasks 4/5: Determine if there is someone who knows the patient's preferences, and who can serve as a surrogate. In this case, the daughter, a first-degree relative, serves as a default informant and surrogate decision maker.

DAUGHTER: Not really. I mean, her doctors made us think she was going to get better.

RESIDENT: We will do everything we can to help her survive, but I must be honest – despite giving her two very strong medicines, her blood pressure is still so low that if it doesn't improve, her organs will fail. Her blood-clotting system is already affected.

DAUGHTER: Well, please do everything you can.

RESIDENT (*nodding*): We absolutely are. But if we are unable to reverse her shock, she will die. Normally, unless you tell us otherwise, if something sudden happens, we will use CPR. If she stops being able to breathe on her own, we can insert a breathing tube and put her on a breathing machine. If her heart stops beating on its own, we can shock her and do chest compressions to try to restart her heart. But these measures will not bring her back to good health – they may simply prolong the dying process, and they are painful. We will try to reverse her shock, but if her lungs or heart stops working, she has a low chance of surviving CPR – about a 2% chance of surviving to leave the hospital. Given the low chance of success, what do you think your mother would want us to do?

DAUGHTER: Well, I know I'd want you to do everything, but...I don't want her to suffer. We had to talk her into having the surgery, she wasn't sure she wanted to go through all that, but she did well.... I don't want her to be in any pain. Is she?

It may seem brutal to describe a patient's condition in such stark terms ("she will die"), but in my experience, people in such situations benefit from simple, clear language. Here the resident spells out what CPR entails and gives a concrete chance of success.

Clearly the resident has an agenda here – to avoid a resuscitation in a patient in whom the chance of success is low. That is not necessarily problematic – in fact, I would argue that not giving families and patients some direction and advice is unfair. Laypersons coping with an emotionally difficult situation with lots of technical issues benefit from a physician laying out the issues. This is where the principle of autonomy must be balanced against beneficence and nonmaleficence.

RESIDENT: We are not giving her pain medicines right now because it would lower her blood pressure even more, and she's already at risk of death from low blood pressure.
(*DAUGHTER starts to cry.*)

RESIDENT (*after 10 seconds of silence*): I am so sorry you're going through this. We want to do everything we can to help your mother. If we can make her better, we will. If we can't, we want to give her as dignified a death as possible.

DAUGHTER (*sobbing*): I just don't know what to do . . .

RESIDENT: Ms. C, for patients in your mother's situation, I think it would be perfectly reasonable to ask for aggressive treatment, but also to ask us *not* to put her through CPR if something sudden should happen. If she doesn't improve soon, it would also be perfectly reasonable for you to ask us to change our focus from treating her shock to keeping her comfortable and focusing on giving her a pain-free, dignified death. She may yet turn around. We'll do our best.

DAUGHTER: Okay.

RESIDENT: I'll have our social worker come talk to you. Please talk to your brother right away and let us know as soon as you can about whether you'd want CPR or if you want to avoid that. We can also discuss changing our goal to keeping her comfortable depending on what happens in the next few hours.

DAUGHER: Okay. Thank you, Doctor.

Total conversation time: 7 minutes.

Ten seconds of silence can feel like an eternity – but it's appropriate to give people space to express their grief. You may find yourself tearing up in such situations. That's human, so if you do, don't sweat it. If continuing the conversation really does not feel right to you, you can always excuse yourself and come back.

Notice how the resident phrases the "no code" option. Families are very burdened by the life-or-death decisions they face with a critically ill loved one who has no advance directive. It is often crucial for doctors to let them know that "no code" options are legitimate, and may even be the medically recommended course. Why? Because these families have to live with their decisions for the rest of their lives. Our medical culture emphasizes autonomy, but taken to an extreme, that can leave bewildered families feeling burdened and isolated. We can relieve their pain by sketching out what we see as reasonable alternatives.

Vignette 2: "Honey, I've Lived a Good Long Time." Mrs. W *is a 62-year-old African American woman with a history of severe asthma who is admitted for progressive dyspnea on exertion. Her intern has just completed the history and physical exam. The patient has had excellent functional status until her symptoms started 6 weeks ago and she has no comorbid conditions.*

Comments

INTERN: Okay, now that we're done with your exam, I've just got one more thing I wanted to ask you about, which I ask all my patients admitted to the hospital. Have you ever talked with your primary doctor about your preferences for CPR, or an advanced directive, or living will?

Notice the intern makes it clear she discusses code status with all her patients, which may reduce any anxiety about the subject.

Task 1: Ask about prior discussion with doctors re: CPR preference.

MRS. W: Living will? No, he's never asked.

INTERN: Okay, well, have you ever talked with anyone about CPR – by which I mean, if you stop breathing on your own, whether you'd want us to put in a breathing tube and help you breathe with a ventilator machine. Or if your heart stopped, would you want CPR with chest compressions or electric shock to try to restart your heart?

Tasks 2/3: Ask about preferences related to intubation and resuscitation.

MRS. W: Honey, I've lived a good long time with this asthma, and if it's my time, it's my time. I don't want to be hooked up to any breathing machines or tubes, and I don't want any shocks.

INTERN: So, it sounds like what you're saying is if something sudden happens to your breathing or your heart, you want us *not* to use aggressive measures to try to reverse it?

Use of restating.

MRS. W: That's right. If the Lord takes me, he takes me.

INTERN: So, we would call that a "DNR/DNI" status.

Intern introduces a bit of jargon that the patient is likely to hear again, if she discusses her code status further.

MRS. W: Okay, if that's what you call it . . . I don't want it.

INTERN: Is there anyone you've spoken to about your preference *not* to have CPR?

Tasks 4/5: Determine if there is someone who knows the patient's preferences, and who can serve as a surrogate.

MRS. W: Well, yes, my goddaughter who lives out of state . . .

INTERN: Can I get her name and number?

MRS. W: Sure. (*Gives the information.*)

INTERN: And if you happen to get so sick that you can't tell us what you want, would you want your goddaughter to help us make decisions for you?

MRS. W: That's right.

INTERN: And, Mrs. W., you've *never* talked to your doctor about your feelings?

Again, the intern here has an agenda – in this case, to probe a patient who is giving a new status of DNR/DNI. Her history and exam did not uncover any obvious signs of depression, the patient is lucid, seems able to give informed consent, and appears to have a rationale for refusing a code. However, she may not actually understand what it is she is refusing, as we'll see. . . . Here the intern clarifies whether Mrs. W. has ever been coded; patients who survive a code have more of an idea of what is involved, and their refusal may come from a more informed position.

MRS. W: No, he's never asked me. He's a wonderful doctor and I know he's trying to get me well, and it's no disrespect to him. But that's my feeling.

INTERN (*nodding*): I understand. But you've never been through CPR before, or had a breathing tube?

MRS. W: No, praise the Lord, I have not. I could never live that way . . .

INTERN: Hmmm. Well, I want to make sure you understand that, with your asthma, the most likely thing that could happen here in the hospital – not that we expect anything to happen, but

The intern gives a basic statistic for the patient's consideration. She doesn't know exactly what the odds of Mrs. W. surviving a code to discharge might be – but that's not crucial. She

if it did – we'd expect that you'd have trouble with your breathing. On average, when people need CPR in the hospital, about 13% of them survive it and are discharged home eventually. But if the trouble was with your breathing, I think your odds of undergoing CPR and eventually going home would be much better than that.

MRS. W: But I don't want to be on a breathing machine.

INTERN: Even if it gets you through a, well, a "rough patch," so you can go home? Even when people with asthma need a breathing tube and a breathing machine to help them when they're very sick, they usually only need it for a few days, sometimes just a few hours. It sounds to me like you think you'd need the breathing machine for a long time.

MRS. W: You mean I wouldn't?

INTERN: Well, there are never any guarantees, but I think the most likely case is that if you did need a breathing machine, you'd need it likely for a few days, not for weeks. Given that, and especially given that you haven't yet had a talk with your doctor about this, I think it'd be wise for us to keep you a "full code" status in case anything happens. At least until you can talk it over more with your doctor?

MRS. W: Well, okay, if you think that's wise . . .

does tell her that it would likely be for an event she'd survive to discharge, and that her odds are better than the average inpatient.

Here the intern uncovers a significant lack of understanding by the patient – she thought being on a ventilator would be a long-term condition. Note the intern doesn't tell her a long intubation won't happen – just that if intubation should occur, for her case it'd likely be short term.

As a student, you may not always know the most likely code scenario for an admitted patient; that takes experience. The main point here is that a patient reporting a DNR status should be probed to make sure that position comes from a full understanding. In this case, it did not, and the intern wisely counseled the patient to maintain "full code" for the time being.

Total conversation time: 6 minutes.

Vignette 3: "What's the Point?" Mr. B *is a 53-year-old Italian American man admitted with an episode of chest pain at rest that occurred 2 hours ago, after 6 months of exertional angina. His chest pain was relieved after a single sublingual nitroglycerin, and his ST-depressions in leads V1–V3 have returned to baseline. He has received aspirin and a beta-blocker. He is being admitted to rule out a non-ST elevation myocardial infarction. His wife is seated next to him. In the history, the student learns that Mr. B has had to take leave from his job as a warehouse supervisor due to his chest pains. She has just finished her initial history and exam.*

STUDENT: Mr. B, thanks for your cooperation. There's just one more thing I want to discuss, which I do with anyone we admit to the hospital. Have you ever talked to your doctors about CPR, or a living will?

MR. B (*seems irritated*): CPR? What? What, you think I'm gonna have a heart attack, here? Is this it?

STUDENT: No, no, Mr. B, not at all — you're not having any chest pain, and your first blood test is negative for a heart attack. But for anybody who comes to the hospital, we want to know, if they should suddenly stop breathing on their own or their heart should stop working, do they want us to use a breathing tube to help them breathe or shocks and chest compressions or strong medicines to help restart their heart.

MR. B: You mean you don't do that *automatically?*

STUDENT: We *always* do it automatically, unless someone tells us they don't want it — that's called "DNAR" status, "Do not attempt resuscitation."

Comments

Task 1: Ask about prior discussion with doctors re: CPR preference.

An example of an unusual bad reaction to introducing the subject of CPR, and how to handle it.

Tasks 2/3: Ask about preferences related to intubation and resuscitation.

MR. B (*seems disgusted*): Yeah, I've seen that on TV.... You know, I'm not good with pain. I don't want any shocks. I don't want any of it.

STUDENT: So, you're telling me you *wouldn't* want a breathing tube if you need help breathing, and you *don't* want CPR to get your heart restarted?

Use of restating.

MR. B: No. I'm sick of this crap. I'm over it. (*Shaking his head . . .*) You know, six months ago, I was healthy . . . healthier than you, even . . .

STUDENT: Mr. B, it sounds to me like your heart disease has really affected your life in a big way. Do you think you might be somewhat depressed? (*Student looks over at the wife, who silently nods her head.*)

MR. B: No, I'm not depressed. I'm just sick of this. Sick of being sick. So, if this is it, if this is the Big One, well, screw it. What's the point?

Here the student appropriately probes a patient giving a new DNR status, and appropriately identifies a complicating factor, which is the possibility of depression – verified by his wife.

STUDENT: Well, listen: I appreciate how you're feeling, but let me tell you a little about CPR. For people who have a sudden event in the hospital, and who have CPR, about 13% of them survive to go home.

Again, observe the use of concrete statistics.

MR. B: That's not very good odds.

STUDENT: Well, in your case, the statistics show that *your* odds are somewhat better than that. If you did have a heart attack, and you did have a bad heart rhythm, we'd see it, and the odds are good we could reverse it.... You've never talked to your doctor about your CPR preference?

MR. B: No, he never asked me.

STUDENT: Well, listen: I know you've said you're not depressed, but even so, I think adjusting to your heart condition has been a big change. I think, until you've had time to talk it over more with your cardiologist, for right now, it's prudent to keep you what we call "full code" status. That means, if you should have a funny heart rhythm, we'll try to reverse it, and that may take shocks, chest compressions, and strong medicines like epinephrine, uh, adrenaline. If you pass out, we may also use a breathing tube to help you breathe, until you can breathe on your own.

MR. B: *Sigh . . .* okay. (*Looks up.*) Okay.

STUDENT: And, I assume you'd want your wife to make decisions if you are not able to tell us yourself?

MR. B: Yeah. (*Turns to wife.*) Honey, make sure they got your phone number . . .

Total conversation time: 4 minutes.

Revisiting Task 1, which never got answered.

Student counsels the patient to hold off on a DNR status until more discussion can occur. She spells out in simple language what CPR will entail.

Tasks 4/5: Determine if there is someone who knows the patient's preferences, and who can serve as a surrogate.

* * *

Personal Finance for the Medical Trainee

Why cover this? A fundamental tenet of *The Nerd's Guide to Pre-Rounding* is that the habits you develop as a student will help or hinder you in residency and your later medical career. It has become clear to me that one important piece of **fostering well-being for future physicians is to call attention to financial literacy** – a quality in dwindling supply among post-Boomers used to living off credit cards. Just as a patient who ignores nagging chest pain may be headed for a major heart attack, a future doctor who ignores his financial picture may wake up down the road stuck with enormous monthly payments, debt loads, or bad credit. You may be blocked from professional or personal dreams.

Why doctors get into trouble. Personal finances lead to strife for many medical professionals. Why? One reason is hubris. Doctors, like many people, are often financially illiterate. However, unlike folks who may be willing to admit their ignorance and address it, doctors may have a hard time admitting they don't know everything. Some seem to think the two letters after their name make them experts in topics beyond medicine, such as business and finance. (If you don't believe this, I can show you an endless list of docs with private practices teetering on the brink of insolvency due to bad financial planning.) Physicians usually are intelligent folks used to mastering all sorts of complicated skills – why should finances be any different?

Doctors all too frequently embody the truism, "Smart people, stupid choices."

Fear is another emotional barrier to tackling finances. Managing money is increasingly complicated and students incurring massive debts can be so paralyzed by anxiety that they don't look the monster straight in the eye. In other words, for many medical professionals, it may not be overconfidence, but lack of confidence.

Finally, simply being overwhelmed by the demands of training can cause significant short-sightedness, by default (and not just about finances – the high rate of divorce among doctors may also be related to emotional myopia). Deferring a plan for finances may be fed by the old saw that "doctors make a lot of money" and so really don't need to worry about making ends meet. Isn't it pretty to think so? Most medical students these days likely have a more realistic outlook about their future income, but nonetheless may not know where to begin.

None of this is helped, for American trainees, by our country's decision in the 1970s to finance the training of physicians through the assumption of enormous personal debt, which helped to fuel the rise of a subspecialist-heavy medical system. This system resulted in trainees having plenty of access to loans and easy money during their training years – racking up debt for decades to come, especially when children and home-buying arrive.

Factor in the dizzying array of grants, loans, and deferments, and you've got a situation that is not only stressful but very confusing. No wonder many future doctors feel like ducking their heads in the sand.

A personal confession. I found the subject of personal finance both boring and bewildering, which is probably why my finances were such a mess when I started medical school. With the help of an incredibly patient financial aid officer, even I, the financially hapless, was able to wend my way through the labyrinth of loans and grants. My partner also helped me get organized – especially by insisting that I put down my credit card debt, the millstone around my neck. If I can do it, you can.

Where to begin? Now, you may be the kind of person who's totally on top of your finances, balance your checkbook every month, and know down to the half penny how much you spent on throat lozenges and lint combs for the past 5 years. If so, bully for you! The advice below is for the rest of us. (Although you may find some of it interesting.)

First, know where your income comes from, and how you're spending it. Many people do not keep a record of their expenditures, which makes it hard to analyze potential trouble spots. If you do not keep track of your income and expenses, your first step is to start doing so. The most basic way to do this: Get a ledger book and start writing down your transactions. Getting receipts for every transaction (including at the ATM) is a good habit that will help with this and will also be helpful if you decide to take deductions on your taxes.

You can also use software to help with tracking expenses and creating budgets. Our family uses a simple Microsoft Excel® spreadsheet. Packages more specific to tracking finances include one called Mvelopes® Personal by In2M (available at www.mvelopes.com), which is web-based. For those who prefer to store their personal information only on a home computer, software packages include Quicken® by Intuit, Microsoft Money®, or MoneyDance®, a simple program downloadable for a free trial (available at www.moneydance.com).

Second, educate yourself. There are several references the total financial illiterate can use to begin his or her education. One excellent resource is Eric Tyson's *Personal Finance for Dummies* (New York: IDG Books). This text gives some very savvy tips that could help you to avoid serious errors in money management. Other texts that may be worthwhile include Beth Kobliner's *Get a*

Financial Life: Personal Finance in Your Twenties and Thirties (New York: Fireside) and *Charles Schwab's Guide to Financial Independence* (New York: Three Rivers Press).

For medical trainees in particular, the Association of American Medical Colleges has an excellent website about the basics of financing a medical education (available at www.aamc.org/ students/financing/start.htm). The site includes a comprehensive review of money management throughout the medical career, "MD2," as well as an email listserv, "Moneymatters," for answering questions on financial aid.

Third, analyze your spending and learn how to save. The better your record-keeping system, the easier it is to do this. Most Americans have a serious problem with overspending – in fact, the average American saves less than 5% of their after-tax income, and a quarter of adults age 35–54 have *not even begun* to save for retirement. (All together now: *Ooof!*) Many people have no regularized savings plan.

Debts come in two forms: Good debts incurred as an investment (e.g., your medical education, which increases your long-term earning potential) and bad debts – namely, debts incurred on consumer items that will not increase in value. An especially pernicious form of bad debt is **credit card debt, which you should consider akin to cancer** – it not only doesn't give back to you, it will actually siphon off future earnings and resources to service the debt. It should be a goal to eliminate your credit card debt as soon as possible and avoid incurring any new debts that cannot be immediately paid off.

Fourth, create an emergency fund. A general guideline is to save 3–6 months of living expenses. This may not be totally practical once you're on a limited income during training, but having a "slush fund" to cover sudden emergencies, e.g., an unexpected car repair, allows you to cope with the unexpected without relying on credit card, –a.k.a.– cancer debt.

Fifth, consider investing. While you may wonder how you can afford to invest while still incurring debt as a student, keep in mind that even a simple savings account is a form of investment (although money market funds may offer better yields). The particularities of choosing forms of investment are beyond the scope of this *Guide*, but I refer you to the references cited for further reading.

Sixth, consider your exposure to risk, and have the right kinds and level of insurance. For many people, the only topic more boring than finance is insurance. Again, as with finances, think about your money as your life energy. Insurance is a form of protection that may make a bad life event survivable rather than devastating.

One essential insurance is **medical** – most students are already covered by their schools, although the coverage may not be totally sufficient if you have special medical concerns. **Disability insurance** is often part of an employment package once you start residency, but likely is not coverage you have as a student. Young people often do not consider **life insurance** unless they have children of their own. Keep in mind, however, that when you finish school and start residency, you will be carrying a substantial educational debt and that debt will be transferred to your dependents or family in the unexpected case of your death. (Grim to think about, isn't it?) The life insurance granted by most residency programs will make just a dent in the total debt load and so extra life insurance would be appropriate. Finally, if you have **assets** such as a home or car, insurance is again prudent. In many cities, affordable **renter's insurance** can cover your belongings in the case of fire or theft – which would be a blessing if you lost your computer, handheld, or other expensive medical books and tools.

Beware the workaholic money trap. The frenetic pace of doctors' lives makes us vulnerable to a terrible blindness. Without

the mental space to step back, take a breath, and set a deliberate
course for our lives, many of us drift, unawares, into long hours
of hard work, high salaries, and even higher levels of consumer
debt incurred spending our money on nice things we *deserve*,
goddammit, because we work so *bloody* hard. And we're often
unhappy.

In an account of their own relationship to money, physicians
Patrick Dunn and Constance Rosson call this story the "conjunction
of material prosperity and social recession," and remark:

> Medical students graduating in 1999 have an average
> $91,000 in loan debt and, like we did, may feel a need for
> delayed gratification. Consumption of high-end homes,
> cars, and travel can lead to an average $200,000 debt for
> practicing physicians. Overworking in today's medical
> environment and servicing a mountain of debt all too often
> lead to stressed relationships and dissatisfaction with
> personal and professional lives.[1]

Another physician, Rick Stahlhut, makes the observation that
doctors who find the subject of money uninteresting may not realize that money is equivalent to life energy:

> If you think money is a boring subject that has nothing to
> do with your ideals and dreams, think again. You trade
> your hours of life for money. If you did not need any
> money, you could give your patients, your family, and
> yourself much more time. Everyone wins if you can find a
> way to need radically less money to be happy, because you
> will regain the flexibility you need to practice medicine
> differently.[2]

---

[1] Dunn PM, Rosson CL, Medicine and money: how much is enough? *West J Med.*
2000;174:10–11.

[2] Stahlhut RW. Making your idealism practical by transforming your relationship
with money. Available: http://my.net-link.net/~stahlhut/escape/idealism.html.

Arguing for a livable life over money may not be a hard sell to Generation X – although that same trait may explain why, compared to the Boomers, the younger generation has an even greater problem with credit card debt. If you are at all intrigued by the comments of the physicians above, check out *Your Money or Your Life: Transforming Your Relationship with Money and Achieving Financial Indepedence* (New York: Penguin Books), by Joe Dominguez and Vicki Robin.

* * *

APPENDIX 8

Using PubMed

What Is PubMed? PubMed is a service of the U.S. National Library of Medicine. It is a search engine that allows you to find articles on biomedical topics from more than 15 million citations dating back to the 1950s. Articles are from journals in the MEDLINE database and other life science journals.

Why use it? On any given day, you will be faced with questions about how to best manage your patients on the wards. To apply evidence-based medicine, you must draw on the literature. PubMed allows you to do this quickly and easily.

How to use it. PubMed is available online though the following link: www.pubmed.com. Often medical schools have a specific link through their library website so that you can link from the PubMed citation to a full-text copy owned by your library.

The PubMed page allows you to type in search terms in an entry field or window. A simple search involves typing terms into the field and hitting "go." For example, let's say our patient has antiretroviral-resistant HIV infection, a condition we don't know much about. If we enter the keywords "antiretroviral," "resistant," and "HIV," and hit go, we will get back more than 800 citations – an impractically high number of articles to find and read.

Narrowing a search using the "limits" page. Let's say we want to limit our search to just *review articles* on antiretroviral-resistant

HIV. Clicking on the "limits" button leads to a separate page where you can narrow your search in various ways. For example, you can limit the field to cover just certain sorts of searches – such as searching by author name or searching only for articles that have our term in the title. In addition to narrowing the field type, you can specify the publication type, e.g., just search for clinical trial results or reviews. You can even limit search results to a specific language, or to cover research on humans or animals, men or women, specific age ranges of subjects, the date of article publication, or how recently the article entered the database. For our example, we could click on "limits" and then on "publication type" and select "review." That gives us more than 220 articles – still a lot. If we then limit the field to "title word," we get down to 4.

Narrowing a search using Boolean modifiers. If you wish, you can have *multiple* field search terms of *different* types (e.g., an article by a certain author that also contains certain title words). Instead of using the limits page, you compose your search terms manually by entering all the terms into the field at the same time, using Boolean modifiers (in all capital letters: AND, NOT, OR) and specifying the field type in brackets. Field types include the title [ti], author [au], specific journal [ta], articles in certain languages [la], or articles of a certain publication type [pt].

Let's say we wanted to find a recent review by Steven G. Deeks on antiretroviral-resistant HIV. Our search field would be:

antiretroviral [ti] AND resistant [ti] AND HIV [ti]
AND deeks sg [au] AND review [pt]

When we hit go, we find one article that fits all those parameters.

Take another example. Let's say our patient has HIV-related lipodystrophy, a condition we've never heard of. If we simply type "lipodystrophy" into the field and hit go, we get more than 2,800 articles. If we go to "limits" and specify publication type as "review," we narrow the result to more than 400. If we further specify that the field cover just title words, we narrow the result to more than 100. We can also specify the language as English, which gets us to 88 results. Note that we could have produced the same search from the start by typing the following into the search field:

lipodystrophy [ti] AND review [pt] AND english [la] = 88 results

We can further narrow our results by looking for articles that are found only in the core medical journals that our library is likely to carry (field term jsubsetaim) or are systematic reviews on a topic (field term systematic [sb]). For example,

lipodystrophy [ti] AND review [pt] AND english [la] AND jsubsetaim

reduces our results from 88 to 12 articles, and

lipodystrophy [ti] AND review [pt] AND english [la] AND systematic [sb]

reduces our 88 results down to 2 citations.

If you wish to search on a specific phrase, such as "HIV-associated nephropathy," enter it with quotation marks:

"HIV-associated nephropathy" = 187 results
"HIV-associated nephropathy" [ti] AND treatment = 34 results

Let's say our patient is being treated with steroids, and we want to know what evidence supports this. We can try

"HIV-associated nephropathy" [ti] AND corticosteroids = 8 results
"HIV-associated nephropathy" [ti] AND corticosteroids [ti] = 2 results

Other approaches would be

"HIV-associated nephropathy" [ti] AND clinical trial [pt] = 2 results
"HIV-associated nephropathy" [ti] AND systematic [sb] = 1 result

If you wish to search on many terms that begin with the same letters, use the star (*) after the common letters. For example, let's say we wanted articles on HIV-related lipo-dystrophy *and* lipo-atrophy. We could type

HIV [ti] and lipo* [ti]

and find articles on both syndromes.

Some of these tips were adapted from notes by Dr. Sanjiv Shah, chief resident, UCSF, 2003–04, who is gratefully acknowledged.

Index